Laboratory Activities for Therapeutic Modalities

Third Edition

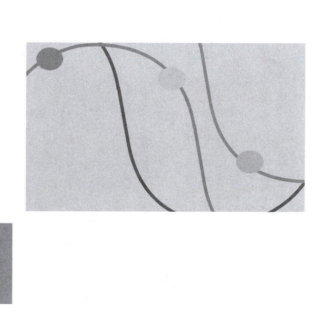

Laboratory Activities for Therapeutic Modalities

Third Edition

MaryBeth Horodyski, EdD, ATC/L

Associate Professor & Research Program Director
Department of Orthopaedics
University of Florida
Gainesville, FL

Chad Starkey, PhD, ATC

Associate Professor, Athletic Training
Northeastern University
Boston, MA

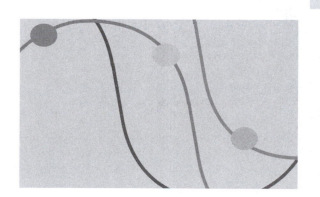

F.A. Davis Company • Philadelphia

F. A. Davis Company
1915 Arch Street
Philadelphia, PA 19103
www.fadavis.com

Printed in the United States of America
Last digit indicates print number: 10 9 8 7 6 5 4 3 2 1
Acquisitions Editor: Christa Fratantoro
Cover Designer: Joan Wendt

As new scientific information becomes available through basic and clinical research, recommended treatments and drug therapies undergo changes. The author(s) and publisher have done everything possible to make this book accurate, up to date, and in accord with accepted standards at the time of publication. The author(s), editors, and publisher are not responsible for errors or omissions or for consequences from application of the book, and make no warranty, expressed or implied, in regard to the contents of the book. Any practice described in this book should be applied by the reader in accordance with professional standards of care used in regard to the unique circumstances that may apply in each situation. The reader is advised always to check product information (package inserts) for changes and new information regarding dose and contraindications before administering any drug. Caution is especially urged when using new or infrequently ordered drugs.

Dedications

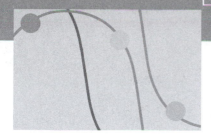

Dedications to the Third Edition:
To Bob, Nicole, Bobby, Jonathan
and the many students
mbh

Warren Zevon
January 24, 1947–September 7, 2003
We'll keep you in our hearts for awhile
cas

Contributors

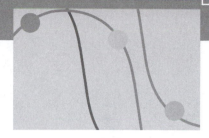

The writing of this text included significant contributions from two exceptional professionals. We would like to thank Traci N. Gearhart, PhD, ATC, and Matthew Morgan, PT, ATC, for their input and countless hours of review.

Traci N. Gearhart, PhD, ATC
Director, Athletic Training Education
Wingate University
Wingate, NC

Matthew Tyrus Morgan, PT, ATC
PhD Student at the University of Florida
Director of Physical Therapy
St. Mary's Center for Sports Medicine and Rehab
Knoxville, TN

Prefaces

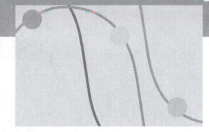

The modalities included in the exercises in this laboratory manual are intended to be used according to the manufacturers' safety and operating recommendations. Contraindications to the use of these modalities must be ascertained and observed.

Preface to the Third Edition

The goals for this edition remain unchanged from those of the first and second editions: to provide students with hands-on activities that illustrate the concepts underlying the use of therapeutic modalities and to promote problem-solving through application of the discovered material. By using the second edition of this lab manual, we saw a need to reorganize the book into units. Each unit begins with basic background information for and contraindications to use of the various modalities. The order of the activities within a unit is intended to build on principles for the use of modalities of similar types.

As with the first and second editions, this manual is designed as an adjunct to a textbook and is not meant to stand alone. Although we have included lists of contraindications to the use of specific modalities at the beginning of each unit, the responsibility to ensure that the activities are conducted safely lies with the instructor.

This edition features a reorganization of the class activities into units to assist students in obtaining concepts of related modalities and treatments in a logical order. The laboratory activities can be conveniently modified by the instructor to incorporate available equipment and different content sequences. We have added more activities, modified others, and updated the questions. Additionally, we moved information presented in the appendices into appropriate units to enhance the concepts being presented within the activity. Lastly, we placed case studies at the end of each unit, thus enhancing practical application of modalities. Students are encouraged to compare and contrast treatments that would be applicable for setting up treatments related to the case studies.

MaryBeth Horodyski
Chad Starkey

Preface to the Second Edition

Our experience with the first edition of this laboratory manual indicates that students are better able to explain concepts after actually experiencing them. Our goals remain the same with this edition: to provide students with hands-on activities that illustrate the concepts underlying the use of therapeutic modalities and to promote problem-solving through application of the discovered material.

As with the first edition, this manual is designed as an adjunct to a textbook and is not meant to stand alone. Although we have included a list of contraindications to the use of specific modalities in Appendix 1, the responsibility to ensure that the activities are conducted safely lies with the instructor.

This edition continues to feature a series of well-structured laboratory activities that can be modified by the instructor to incorporate available equipment and different content sequences. We have added some activities, modified others, and updated the questions and answers following each to reflect the most current research findings.

We have also added a Universal Skill Assessment Instrument (following the case studies) that allows evaluation of the actual modality application. This tool can be used in conjunction with the case studies or as a student is practicing actual modality application.

Sara D. Brown
Chad Starkey

Preface to the First Edition

After many combined years between us of teaching therapeutic modalities, we found a need for structured laboratory activities beyond the rote setup and application of the equipment. Too often students were becoming technicians rather than clinicians. We also found a secondary need to expose the student to the physical sensations and the physiological effects of the energy delivered by therapeutic modalities, reinforcing the didactic segment of our courses. This manual represents our combined efforts to improve the students' laboratory experience with therapeutic modalities.

This laboratory manual is designed to be an adjunctive tool for most of the existing textbooks on therapeutic modalities and should not be considered a stand-alone text on this topic. While we have included contraindications for each of the modalities used (Appendix I), the ultimate responsibility for the safe setup and application rests with the students and their instructors.

While structured procedures are described for each of the activities, they may be modified by the instructor to make use of the available equipment and fit the educational level of the students. Depending on the experience of the student, this laboratory manual provides avenues for incorporating therapeutic exercise into many of the activities, exercises, and case studies. The quasi-experimental design of the activities allows the integration of statistical analysis. Before the beginning of the class, the instructor should refer to Appendix A for an explanation of the equipment used in measuring skin temperature.

Each activity is followed by a series of discussion questions. A brief explanation and rationale for the correct response appears in Appendix E. Perforated pages are provided so that the results of the class activities and exercises can be submitted at the instructor's request.

Copies of the grids for each activity are provided in Appendix H. The intent of these grids is to allow the student to repeat an exercise. Please avoid the temptation to copy these for mass distribution.

The manual concludes with a series of case studies. After much deliberation we decided to include only a list of the problems that should be surmised from each case (Appendix G). The wide range of methodologies and ideologies surrounding treatment options made even an effort to create a "correct" response dubious at best.

Chad Starkey
Sara D. Brown

Contents

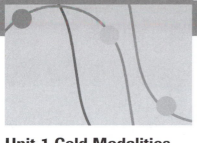

Cold Modalities

Background and Discussion

The most frequently used modalities are cold modalities. Cryotherapy is the application of cold modalities that have a temperature range between 32°F and 65°F (0°C and 18°C). During cryotherapy, heat is removed from the body and absorbed by the cold modality until the temperatures are equal. The body's response to cold modalities can be seen using many different physiological parameters. Changes may be noted through nervous system responses, vascular changes, and cellular changes, specifically decreased cellular metabolism. In most cases, orthopaedic injuries may be treated with cold modalities with little risk of adverse reactions.

The magnitude of skin temperature decrease is directly related to the temperature of the applied modality, the temperature of the tissues, the duration of application, and the conductivity of the tissue being cooled. Because the heat transfer is occurring via conduction (or evaporation, in the case of the vapocoolant spray), the greater the temperature decrease, the greater the transfer of thermal energy and subsequent cooling of the skin. For the benefits of cold to occur, the skin temperature must be decreased to around 57°F.[1]

Generally, however, cold modalities are used to affect changes deep within the tissues. How does a drop in surface temperature correspond with deep tissue changes? The correlation between the decrease in skin temperature and the decrease in intra-articular temperature has been calculated to be 0.65.[2] However, the conductivity of the tissues being treated and the duration of the cold application must be considered. Tissues with a low water content, such as fat, are good insulators and do not allow the transfer of thermal energy. (Witness the blubber-protected whale swimming comfortably in the cold ocean.) By comparison, muscle tissue with its relatively high water content is a good conductor and allows the energy to be absorbed and transmitted to deeper tissues. The application duration also influences the depth of penetration. Whereas it does not take long to evoke superficial changes in temperature, targeting deep tissues requires a longer application time.

A typical ice application protocol following acute injury is 30 minutes on/90 minutes off, based on tissue rewarming times for a stationary patient. Movement (e.g., showering, dressing, returning home) necessitates more frequent application, especially during the period immediately following injury.[3]

It is commonly reported that four distinct sensory phases will be experienced during cold application: cold, burning, aching, and analgesia.[5] The degree of vulnerability of different nerves to cold application accounts for the changes in sensation experienced as the cold treatment progresses. Unmyelinated, small-diameter, superficial pain nerves are stimulated before the larger, myelinated, and deeper nerves. The initial pain experienced during ice immersion results from stimulation of pain-carrying nerves. As the exposure to the cold continues, the perception of pain decreases because of the decrease in nerve conduction velocity of these nerves and the subsequent stimulation of sensory nerves. True anesthesia (the inability to transmit nerve impulses) has not been proved to occur during ice immersion.[6]

Most people find the first application of ice painful. The sensations the patient is told to expect influence the perception of the cold treatment. In general, patients given descriptors of sensations to expect experience less overall pain during the treatment.[7]

A typical scenario for an injured athlete is to apply ice to the injured area and to return to activity. Some have argued that this may actually place the athlete in danger of further injury secondary to changes attributed to cold (e.g., slowed nerve conduction velocity). Research has indicated that eccentric force production[10] and knee joint position sense[11] are not affected following cold treatment, although other research has not been as definitive. Results of functional testing following cold immersion are equivocal, with one study finding no negative effects demonstrated in the shuttle run and 6-meter hop but a decrease in vertical jump height.[9]

The fear of frostbite causes many clinicians to apply an insulator such as an Ace wrap or towel between the cold modality and the skin. Does this practice reduce the effectiveness of the treatment? Because a relationship exists between reduction in skin temperature and the temperature reduction in tissues underlying the treatment area, by measuring the reduction in surface temperature under different treatment conditions, we can ascertain the relative effectiveness of different treatment techniques.

The risk of frostbite depends on the temperature of the applied modality, the duration of the treatment, and the neurovascular properties of the area being treated. Cold modalities that use frozen water, crushed ice packs, ice massage, or ice immersion have a decreased risk of tissue damage because of the melting of the ice. When these cold modalities are applied to a body part that has intact nervous and vascular function for the recommended treatment duration (10 to 30 minutes), the chance of frostbite is virtually nonexistent, even when the modality is applied directly to the skin. However, when a modality such as a reusable cold pack (which is water mixed with antifreeze and stored at temperatures well below the freezing point) is used or when cold modalities are applied for an extended duration, the chance of frostbite increases.

For this reason, reusable cold packs must be applied with a wet insulating medium. The risk of frostbite also increases when cold is applied to areas with poor neurovascular function. When using cold modalities on individuals with conditions such as peripheral vascular disease, the skin must be insulated and the individual closely monitored.

Contraindications

- Cardiac or respiratory involvement
- Uncovered open wounds
- Circulatory insufficiency
- Cold allergy
- Anesthetic skin
- Raynaud's phenomenon
- Presence of regenerating peripheral nerves

Skin Temperature Decrease

■ Objective

To evaluate the relative effectiveness of various cold modalities in decreasing the skin surface temperature and the duration of the decrease.

■ Materials Needed

- Surface temperature gauge (Appendix A)
- Various methods of delivering cold (crushed ice bag, ice immersion bucket in the range of 45° to 55°F, ice massage cup, reusable cold pack, instant cold pack, vapocoolant spray)
- Timing device

■ Procedures

1. Using the surface temperature gauge, record the baseline skin temperature of the surface area to be evaluated. Record this reading on the chart provided. Using a straight-edge, mark this line across the grid. This is your baseline.
2. Apply the cold modality to the body part in the prescribed manner for a total of 10 minutes, with the exception of the vapocoolant spray, which should be applied as recommended by the manufacturer.

3. OPTIONAL: If an electronic skin temperature probe is available, the changes in skin temperature during certain types of cold application can be measured and recorded in 2-minute intervals. Cover the probe end to limit influence from the modality itself.
4. On removing the modality, measure the skin temperature, and record this at the "10-minute" mark on the chart.
5. Every 2 minutes, remeasure the skin temperature, and make the proper notation on the chart.
6. Repeat Step 5 until the skin temperature returns to the baseline value or the 20-minute post-treatment period has expired.
7. Using a different body area on a different extremity, repeat Steps 1 through 6 with another cold modality.
8. On completion of the activity, plot the changes in skin temperature resulting from each modality.

■ Notes

- This activity may be performed using more than one modality at once, provided each is applied to a separate body area.
- A layer of wet insulation must be used when applying reusable cold packs to the body.

Skin Temperature Decrease

Name: _____   Date: _____

Subject(s): _____

Modality used _____

	Baseline	During Application				
	0	2	4	6	8	10
Skin temperature						

	Baseline	Post-Application									
	0	2	4	6	8	10	12	14	16	18	20
Skin temperature											

Modality used _____

	Baseline	During Application				
	0	2	4	6	8	10
Skin temperature						

	Baseline	Post-Application									
	0	2	4	6	8	10	12	14	16	18	20
Skin temperature											

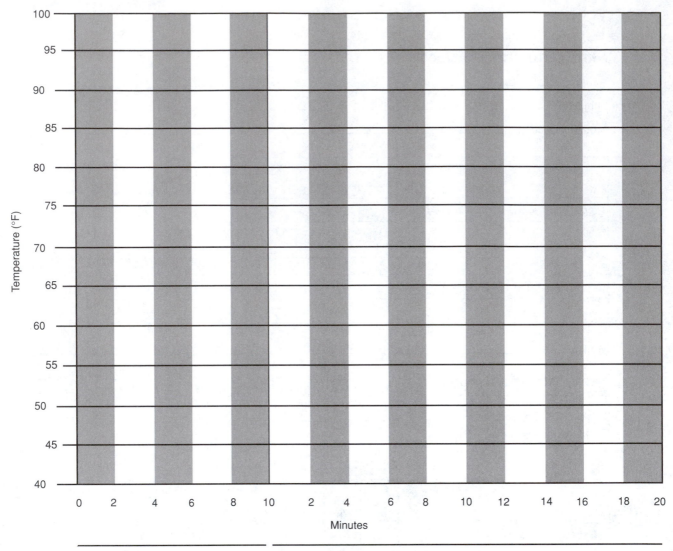

Skin Temperature During Treatment   Skin Temperature Post-Treatment

Using the key below, on graph paper or a spreadsheet program, plot the changes in skin temperature for the modalities used for the laboratory activity. Use this graph to answer the Activity Questions.

Labeling Key	
○ Crushed Ice Bag	■ Reusable Cold Pack
● Ice Immersion	△ Instant Cold Pack
□ Ice Massage	▲ Vapocoolant Spray

■ **Activity Questions**

1. Of the different types of cold application used, which had the greatest change in surface temperature? Why?

2. If cold acts as a vasoconstrictor, why does the skin turn red during cold application?

3. Based on the skin temperature changes, which method would you assume had the least depth of penetration? How would this influence your selection of a cold modality?

Effects of Insulating Media and Compression on Skin Temperature Decrease

Objective

To determine the effect that various insulating media and circumferential compression have on the rate and magnitude of skin temperature decrease.

Materials Needed

- Crushed ice pack
- Wet elastic wrap
- Thermometer
- Damp terry-cloth towel
- Dry terry-cloth towel
- Dry elastic wrap
- Timing device

Procedures

1. Using the surface temperature gauge, record the baseline skin temperature of the area to be treated. Record this reading on the chart provided and, using a straight-edge, mark this line across the grid.
2. Cover the area to be treated with an insulating medium, and apply the crushed ice pack for a total of 10 minutes. If an electronic skin temperature probe is available, the changes in skin temperature during the cold application may be measured and recorded in 2-minute intervals.
3. On removing the modality, measure the skin temperature, and record this at the "10-minute" mark on the chart.
4. Every 2 minutes, remeasure the skin temperature, and make the proper notation on the chart.
5. Repeat Step 4 until the skin temperature returns to the baseline value.
6. Using a different body area on a different extremity, repeat Steps 1 through 5 until all of the following conditions have been tested:
   - Wet elastic wrap between the ice and the skin
   - Damp towel between the ice and the skin
   - Dry towel between the ice and the skin
   - Ice directly to the skin secured with a compressive wrap
7. On completion of the activity, plot the changes in skin temperature resulting from each condition. Transpose onto this grid the skin temperature decrease for a crushed ice pack (with no barrier and no compression) obtained during Activity 1–1.

Notes

- This activity may be performed using more than one cold treatment at once, provided each is applied to a separate body area.
- If limited time precludes each student from experiencing each condition, assign specific conditions to different students, and adjust the data to a common baseline for plotting purposes.
- If time permits, add the condition of using an electrode between the ice and the skin.

Effects of Insulating Media and Compression on Skin Temperature Decrease

Name: _____   Date: _____

Subject(s): _____

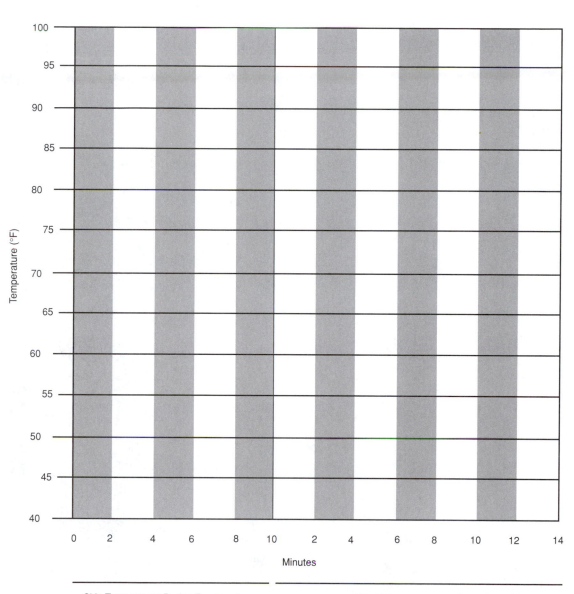

Skin Temperature During Treatment

Skin Temperature Post-Treatment

Labeling Key	
○ Wet elastic wrap	■ Ice and compression
● Damp towel	△ Ice no compression
□ Dry towel	

Activity Questions

1. Considering the relationship between tissue water content and conductivity discussed in Activity 1–1, under which condition would you expect the greatest surface temperature change? Explain your response.

2. What can you conclude about the effectiveness of ice application using different insulating media?

3. Compare the temperature change produced during the compressed ice bag condition with your other findings. What precautions can you conclude from this information?

Cold: Changes in Heart Rate, Blood Pressure, and Skin Appearance

Objective

To determine what, if any, changes occur in heart rate, blood pressure, and skin appearance from the application of various cold modalities.

Materials Needed

- Timing device
- Blood pressure cuff and stethoscope
- Various methods of delivering cold:
  Crushed ice bag (large)
  Ice immersion bucket (temperature range 45°F to 55°F)
  Cold whirlpool

Procedures

1. Using the right arm, determine the subject's pulse rate and blood pressure. To monitor the pulse, palpate the radial artery at the anterior wrist for 15 seconds, and multiply that value by 4 to calculate the beats per minute. Record heart rate on the chart provided. Using the blood pressure cuff and stethoscope, record the baseline blood pressure. Record this reading on the chart provided. Record information related to skin appearance (color, dry, moist, etc).
2. Apply the cold modality to the body part in the prescribed manner for a total of 10 minutes.
3. During the 10 minutes of application, measure and record blood pressure and heart rate every 2 minutes.
4. At minute 5, record information related to skin appearance.
5. Remove the cold modality, and record information on skin appearance.
6. Remeasure blood pressure and heart rate at 2-minute intervals for 10 minutes after removal of the cold modality, and make the proper notation on the chart.
7. Using a different body area on a different extremity, repeat Steps 1 through 6 with a different modality. Students may also try immersing the lower body by standing or sitting in a cold whirlpool.
8. On completion of the activity, plot on graph paper (or use a computer spreadsheet program) the changes in blood pressure and heart rate resulting from each modality.

Cold: Changes in Heart Rate, Blood Pressure, and Skin Appearance

Name: _____ Date: _____

Subject(s): _____

Modality used _____

	Baseline	During Application					Post-Application				
	0	2	4	6	8	10	2	4	6	8	10
Heart rate											
Systolic blood pressure											
Diastolic blood pressure											

Skin Appearance
Pretreatment _____

During application (minute 5) _____

End of application (minute 10) _____

Post-application (minute 10) _____

Modality used _____

	Baseline	During Application					Post-Application				
	0	2	4	6	8	10	2	4	6	8	10
Heart rate											
Systolic blood pressure											
Diastolic blood pressure											

Skin Appearance
Pretreatment _____

During application (minute 5) _____

End of application (minute 10) _____

Post-application (minute 10) _____

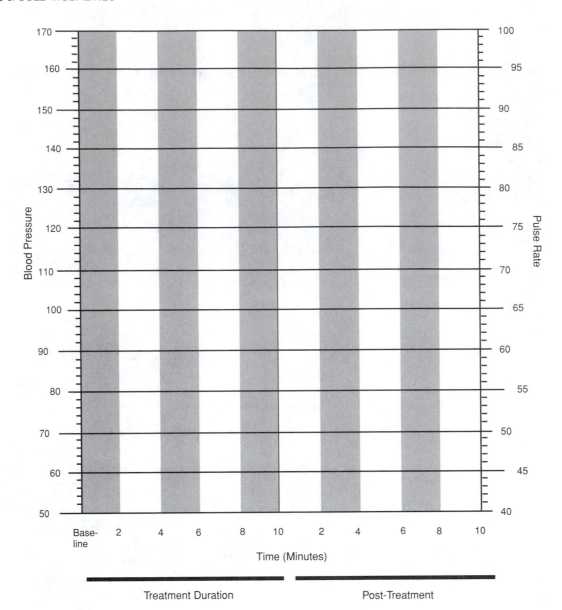

Using the key below, on graph paper plot the changes in heart rate, systolic and diastolic blood pressure recorded for the modalities used for the laboratory activity. Use different colored lines for the different modalities tested. Use this graph to answer the Activity Questions

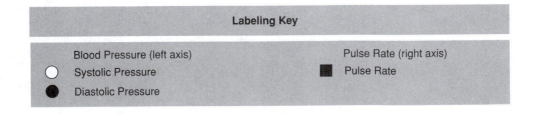

Activity Questions

1. When using a cold modality, is it important to establish the cardiovascular health status of your patient prior to use of the modality? Why?

2. Which of the modalities used demonstrated the greatest changes in blood pressure and heart rate? Why?

3. Was there a difference between cold modalities with respect to return to normal blood pressure and heart rate? Why might this occur?

Pain Perception During Ice Immersion

Objective

To gain an understanding of the sensations related to cold application, acquire knowledge in the use of pain scales, and ascertain the effect of Neoprene® toe caps in changing the comfort level of ice immersion.

Materials Needed

- Ice immersion bucket
- Numerical Rating Scale
- Neoprene toe cap
- Timing device
- Thermometer for measuring the temperature of the immersion

Description of the Numerical Rating Scale

Several simple pain rating scales may be used to measure an individual's pain objectively. The Visual Analog Scale (VAS) employs a 10-cm line describing a continuum between "no pain," at the low end and the "worst pain imaginable," at the high end (Fig. 1–1). Subjects mark a point on the line that best represents the current level of pain they are experiencing. The patient's pain rating is determined by measuring in centimeters from the right-hand border of the line to the mark. The disadvantage of this system is that the lack of coordinates decreases the specificity of rating.[4] The advantage of this system is found in the use of words to describe the extremes of pain.

The Numerical Rating Scale (NRS) uses a numerical scale ranging from "0," representing "no pain," to "10," representing the "worst pain imaginable." Subjects are then asked to circle the whole number between 0 and 10 that best represents their current pain level. The advantage of this system lies in the use of graded intervals to measure pain intensity. The disadvantage is in the lack of descriptors at the extremes. For this workbook we have merged the two scales, combining the intervals of the NRS with the descriptors in the VAS (Fig. 1–2).

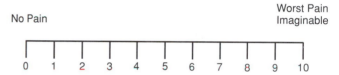

No Pain / Worst Pain Imaginable

0 1 2 3 4 5 6 7 8 9 10

Figure 1–2.   Combined VAS and NRS scale.

Procedures for Using the NRS

Subjects view the modified NRS and circle the number best describing their current level of pain. It is customary to circle only a whole number. Therefore, circling "7" is an appropriate response, whereas marking the position on the grid representing "7.5" is not appropriate. When multiple measures are being made, the subject is not permitted to view the previous response. Once a scale is marked, it should be covered with a piece of paper until the exercise is completed.

Procedures

1. Fill an immersion bucket with water, and add ice to decrease the temperature to between 50°F and 55°F.
2. Inform the subject that this activity will cause a moderate amount of pain. If the pain becomes too great or if the subject experiences lightheadedness, discontinue the activity. Do not give further descriptive information regarding expected sensations.
3. Instruct the subject to immerse a leg in the bucket. For consistency, do not permit talking among the participants for the duration of the experiment.

No Pain / Worst Pain Imaginable

Figure 1–1.   Visual Analog Scale.

4. After 1 minute, have the subject circle the number on the modified NRS that best describes the level of pain experienced.
5. Cover this and future responses so that the subject cannot see the previous responses.
6. Repeat the pain assessment every 2 minutes for the duration of the treatment.
7. After 11 minutes have passed, instruct the subject to remove the foot from the immersion. Have the subject continue to use the scale every 2 minutes until no pain is reported.
8. Plot the changes in perception of cold sensation over time on the accompanying worksheet.
9. Repeat this activity with the same subject using the opposite leg. However, this time have the subject cover the toes with a Neoprene® toe cap.

Pain Perception During Ice Immersion

Name: _____   Date: _____

Subject(s): _____

1 Minute into Immersion

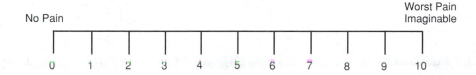

3 Minutes into Immersion

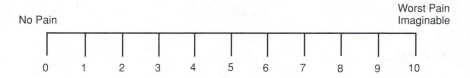

5 Minutes into Immersion

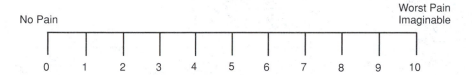

7 Minutes into Immersion

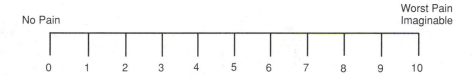

9 Minutes into Immersion

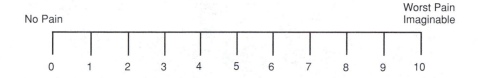

11 Minutes into Immersion

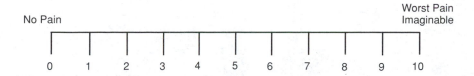

2 Minutes Post-Immersion

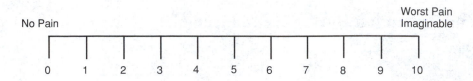

4 Minutes Post-Immersion

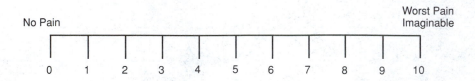

6 Minutes Post-Immersion

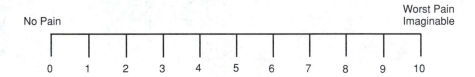

8 Minutes Post-Immersion

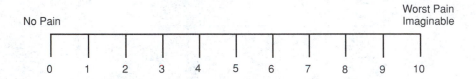

10 Minutes Post-immersion

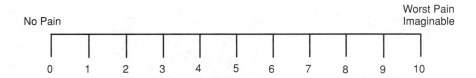

Plot of Pain Perception Over Time

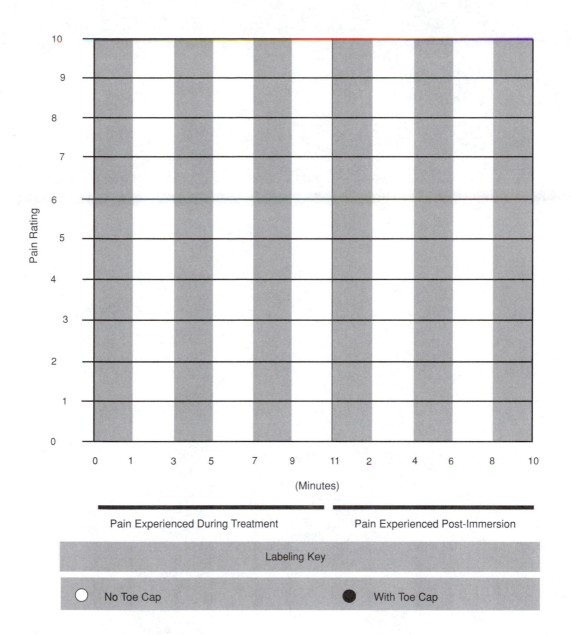

Pain Experienced During Treatment   **Pain Experienced Post-Immersion**

Labeling Key

○ No Toe Cap   ● With Toe Cap

Activity Questions

1. Did your foot and ankle become numb during the immersion? Why or why not?

2. Where was your pain primarily located? Did the use of the toe cap change your perception of pain? Why or why not?

3. Do you think your response to the cold immersion would differ if you were to perform this exercise repeatedly over a week and remeasure perception during the last session? Why or why not?

The Effects of Cooling on Speed, Agility, and Proprioception

Objective

To determine the effect that cooling the foot, ankle and lower leg has on agility, speed, and proprioception.

Materials Needed

- Ice bath (50°F to 55°F)
- Timing device
- Tape (to mark lines for shuttle run and vertical jump)

Description of Measurement of Agility, Speed, and Proprioception

Functional performance has been measured using a variety of methods, including shuttle runs, vertical jumps, carioca maneuvers, cocontraction tests, and hopping tests.[8,9] For this exercise, we recommend the shuttle run (to capture speed abilities), single-leg vertical jump (to capture explosive abilities), and a single-limb balance for time (to capture proprioceptive abilities). Subjects should wear athletic shoes for each event and be given a chance to practice and familiarize themselves with the activity prior to actual testing.

For the shuttle run, place two lines on the floor 6 yards apart. Subjects, standing behind one of the lines, are instructed to run as quickly as possible to the next line, touch it with a foot, turn, and return to the starting line. This sequence is repeated (Fig. 1–3).

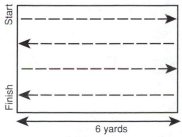

Figure 1–3.   Line marking for shuttle run.

The least expensive way to conduct the single-leg vertical jump is simply to tape a tape measure to the wall from a set height. Commercial devices (e.g., Vertec) are also available and alleviate the problem of the wall. To conduct the test, the subject should first determine which leg is most comfortable for take-off. (This also determines which leg will be submerged.) Next, determine the subject's standing reach. Finally, instruct the subject to stand on the preferred leg and, leading with the arms, to jump as high as possible, touching the wall at the apex of the jump. The difference between the standing reach and the height of the jump constitutes the score.

To assess single-limb balance, time the duration that the subject can stand on the test limb (arms out to the sides) without touching any supporting surface with the arms or opposite limb. For safety purposes, a wall should be within the subject's reach.

Procedures

1. Establish baseline data for each subject in each test, and record the results.
2. Instruct the subject to immerse the preferred take-off leg in the bucket for 10 minutes. (For consistency, each subject should submerge the same amount of leg.)
3. Instruct the subject to dry off quickly and to put on shoes after the immersion. Subjects should perform a brief calf-stretch before the functional testing.
4. Repeat the functional testing, varying the testing sequence among the subjects. Record the results.
5. OPTIONAL: A Student's t-Test can be used to identify statistically significant differences between the pre-test and post-test scores on each of the three functional tests. The t-Test can be conducted using commercially available software such as Excel, SPSS-PC, or MiniTab.

Note: Subjects with a recent history of lower extremity injury should not participate in this activity.

The Effects of Cooling on Speed, Agility, and Proprioception

Name: _____   Date: _____

Subject(s): _____

Subject	Shuttle Run (Time in Seconds)			Single-Leg Jump (Height in Inches)*			Single-Leg Balance (Time in Seconds)		
	Pre-Test	Post-Test	Diff.	Pre-Test	Post-Test	Diff.	Pre-Test	Post-Test	Diff.
NET CHANGE									

*Subtract the standing reach height from the jump height to obtain the measurement value.

■ Activity Questions

1. What does a comparison of pre-test and post-test results reveal? To what do you attribute any differences? What might explain the results of the functional testing study described above?

2. Based on your results from Activity 1–1, Skin Temperature Decrease, how do you think your results would change if an ice bag had been used instead of cold immersion? Justify your response.

3. Is the information derived from this type of research clinically relevant in the management of acute athletic injuries?

On completion of the activities for Unit 1, review the following case studies to enhance practical application of cold modalities.

1. You are preparing to treat a patient for a quadriceps contusion. This is the first time you have treated this individual. What modality would you use? Why? What contraindications would you need to address with your choice of modality?

2. A swimmer reports to the athletic training clinic with a complaint of spasm in her rhomboids. She awoke with the spasm and must compete in her conference meet today. What modality would you choose and why?

3. During the first half of a women's field hockey game, one of the players is hit with a stick on the anterior aspect of the shin. She has no signs of a fracture; the area is slightly discolored and has minimal swelling. She has full ankle and knee ROM and strength. The athlete wants to return to the game; what would your treatment be, and would you allow her to return to the game? Why or why not? Did the results of Activity 1–5 have any influence on your decision?

Superficial Heat Modalities

Background and Discussion

With the application of superficial heating agents, the surface temperature increase correlates to the subcutaneous temperature increase. The extent of the temperature increase depends on the treatment duration, conductive qualities of the tissue, and the conductive qualities of the heating agent. In general, heat does not penetrate as deeply as cold because the increased blood flow acts to dissipate the heat.

Contraindications

- Acute injuries
- Impaired circulation
- Poor thermal regulation
- Anesthetic areas
- Existing fever
- Malignancies
- Cardiac insufficiency
- Extremely old adults and children younger than 4 years
- Pregnancy

Superficial Heat: Skin Temperature Increase

Objective

To determine the relative effectiveness of various heat modalities in increasing the skin surface temperature and the duration of the increase.

Materials Needed

- Surface temperature gauge
- Timing device
- Various methods of delivering heat:
  - Moist heat pack
  - Paraffin
  - Warm whirlpool/warm water immersion
  - Infrared lamp
- Topical counterirritant

Procedures

1. Using the surface temperature gauge, record the baseline skin temperature of the area to be treated. Record this reading on the chart provided.
2. Apply the heat modality to the body part in the prescribed manner for a total of 10 minutes.
3. OPTIONAL: If an electronic skin temperature probe is available and the particular modality makes it feasible, measure the changes in skin temperature during the heat application, and record the findings in 2-minute intervals. Insulate the side of the probe exposed to the heat pack to limit influence from the modality itself. Failure to insulate the probe may result in temperature recording that reflects the average of the skin-modality interface.
4. On removing the modality, measure the skin temperature, and record this at the "10-minute" mark on the chart.
5. Remeasure the skin temperature at 2-minute intervals, and make the proper notation on the chart.
6. Repeat Step 5 until the skin temperature returns to the baseline value or the 20-minute post-treatment period has expired.
7. Using a different body area on a different extremity, repeat Steps 1 through 6 with a different modality.
8. On completion of the activity, plot the changes in skin temperature resulting from each modality.
9. Students are encouraged to enter data into a spreadsheet and plot it to view temperature changes graphically.

Notes

1. This activity may be performed using more than one modality at once, provided each is applied to a separate body area.
2. This laboratory activity can be modified by plotting skin temperature changes using different thicknesses of insulation for moist heat packs.

Superficial Heat: Skin Temperature Increase

Name: _____ Date: _____

Subject(s): _____

Modality used _____

	Baseline	During Application				
	0	2	4	6	8	10
Skin temperature						

	Baseline	Post-Application									
	0	2	4	6	8	10	12	14	16	18	20
Skin temperature											

Modality used _____

	Baseline	During Application				
	0	2	4	6	8	10
Skin temperature						

	Baseline	Post-Application									
	0	2	4	6	8	10	12	14	16	18	20
Skin temperature											

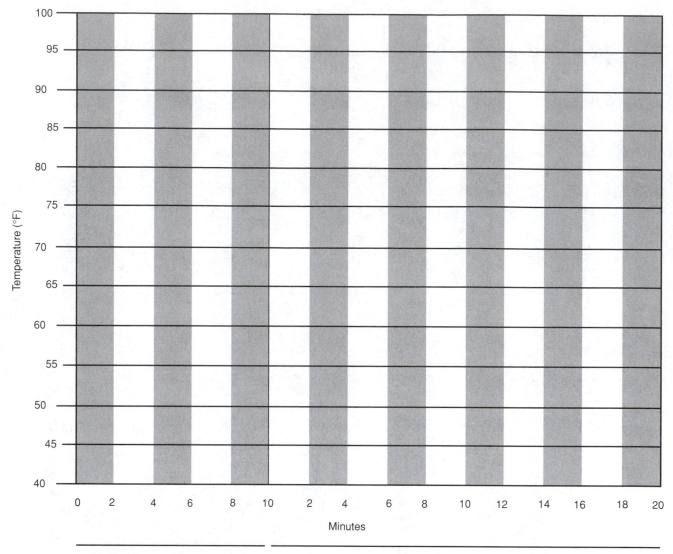

Skin Temperature During Treatment   Skin Temperature Post-Treatment

Using the key below, on graph paper or a spreadsheet program, plot the changes in skin temperature for the modalities used for the laboratory activity. Use this graph to answer the Activity Questions.

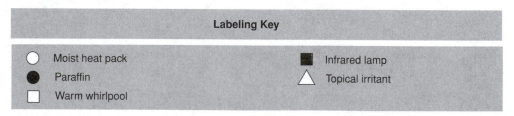

Labeling Key

○ Moist heat pack   ■ Infrared lamp
● Paraffin   △ Topical irritant
□ Warm whirlpool

Activity Questions

1. Which of the modalities used demonstrated the greatest skin temperature increase? Why?

2. Compare the findings of the skin temperature increase and the skin temperature decrease exercises. Which condition demonstrated the longer time for return to normal skin temperature? Why does this occur?

Superficial Heat: Changes in Heart Rate, Blood Pressure, and Skin Appearance

Objective

To determine what, if any, changes occur in heart rate, blood pressure, and skin appearance as the result of application of various heat modalities.

Materials Needed

- Watch with a second hand
- Timing device
- Blood pressure cuff and stethoscope
- Various methods of delivering heat:
  - Moist heat pack
  - Paraffin
  - Warm whirlpool/warm water immersion
  - Infrared lamp
  - Topical counterirritant

Procedures

1. Using the right arm, determine the subject's pulse rate and blood pressure. To monitor the pulse, palpate the radial artery at the anterior wrist for 15 seconds, and multiply that value by 4 to get the beats per minute.

Record heart rate on the chart provided. Using the blood pressure cuff and stethoscope, record baseline blood pressure. Record this reading on the chart provided. Record information related to skin appearance (color, dry, moist, etc).

2. Apply the heat modality to the body part in the prescribed manner for a total of 10 minutes.
3. During the 10 minutes of application, measure and record blood pressure and heart rate every 2 minutes.
4. At minute 5, record information related to skin appearance.
5. Remove the heat modality, and record information on skin appearance.
6. Remeasure blood pressure and heart rate at 2-minute intervals for 10 minutes after removal of the heat modality, and make the proper notation on the chart.
7. Using a different body area on a different extremity, repeat Steps 1 through 6 with a different modality. Students may also try immersing the lower body by standing or sitting in a warm whirlpool.
8. On completion of the activity, plot on graph paper or a computer spreadsheet program the changes in blood pressure and heart rate resulting from each modality.

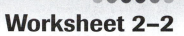

Superficial Heat: Changes in Heart Rate, Blood Pressure, and Skin Appearance

Name: _____   Date: _____

Subject(s): _____

Modality used _____

	Baseline	During Application					Post-Application				
		2	4	6	8	10	2	4	6	8	10
Heart rate											
Systolic blood pressure											
Diastolic blood pressure											

Skin Appearance

Pretreatment _____

During application (minute 5) _____

End of application (minute 10) _____

Post-application (minute 10) _____

Modality used _____

	Baseline	During Application					Post-Application				
		2	4	6	8	10	2	4	6	8	10
Heart rate											
Systolic blood pressure											
Diastolic blood pressure											

Skin Appearance

Pretreatment _____

During application (minute 5) _____

End of application (minute 10) _____

Post-application (minute 10) _____

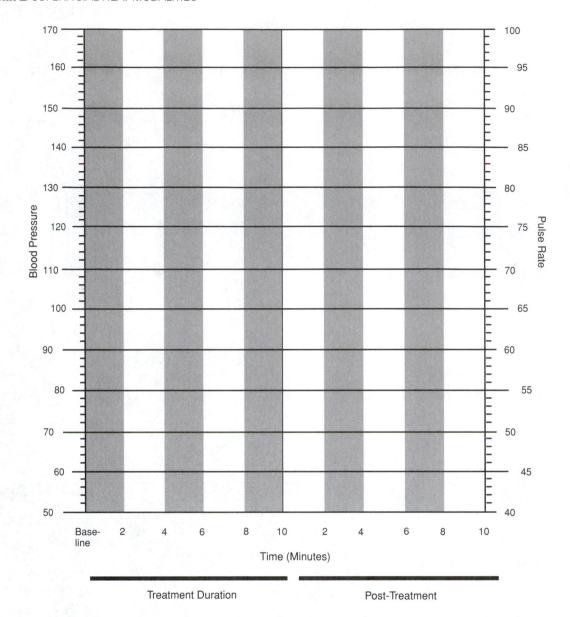

Time (Minutes)

Treatment Duration   Post-Treatment

Using the key below, plot on graph paper the changes in heart rate and systolic and diastolic blood pressure recorded for the modalities used for the laboratory activity. Use different-colored lines for the different modalities tested. Use this graph to answer the Activity Questions.

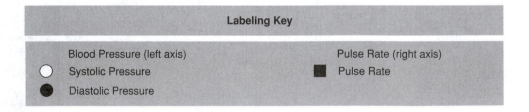

Labeling Key

Blood Pressure (left axis)	Pulse Rate (right axis)
○ Systolic Pressure	■ Pulse Rate
● Diastolic Pressure	

■ Activity Questions

1. When preparing to use a superficial heat modality, is it important to establish the cardiovascular health status of your patient prior to use of the modality? Why?

2. Which of the modalities used demonstrated the greatest changes in blood pressure and heart rate? Why?

3. Was there a difference between heat modalities with respect to return to normal blood pressure and heart rate? Why might this occur?

Superficial Heat: Paraffin Bath

Objective

To determine the effects of paraffin application on joint range of motion (ROM).

Materials Needed

- Paraffin bath
- Plastic bags
- Towels
- Athletic tape
- Goniometer

Procedures

1. Take premeasurements of joint ROM.
2. Choose one of the following methods.
   a) Immersion bath
      i)   Clean the area to be treated.
      ii) Instruct the subject to avoid touching the sides and bottom of the heating unit because burns may result.
      iii) Instruct the subject to not move the body part while in the paraffin. Cracking of the wax will allow fresh hot wax to touch the skin, increasing the risk of burns.
      iv) Have the subject dip the body part into the paraffin and remove it. Allow this coat to dry. (Paraffin will turn a dull shade of white.)
      v)   Dip the extremity into the wax 6 to 12 more times; allow the wax to dry between dips.
      vi) After the final time, the patient then places the body part back into the paraffin for the duration of the treatment. (15–20 minutes)
      vii) After the treatment, remove the hardened paraffin, and return it to the unit for reheating, or discard.
   b) Pack (Glove) Method
      i)   Clean the area to be treated.
      ii) Have the subject dip the body part into the paraffin and remove it. Allow this coat to dry. (Paraffin will turn a dull shade of white.)
      iii) Continue to dip and remove the body part in the wax 6 to 12 times.
      iv) After the final application of wax withdrawal, cover the extremity with a plastic bag, aluminum foil, or wax paper. Wrap and secure the area with a terry-cloth towel for the remainder of the treatment. (15–20 minutes)
      v)   If indicated, the body part may be elevated.
      vi) After the treatment, remove the hardened paraffin, and return it to the unit for reheating, or discard.
3. Repeat ROM measurements.

Note: Assessing temperature changes by taking pre- and post-treatment skin temperatures may enhance this activity.

Superficial Heat: Paraffin Bath

Name: _____   Date: _____

Subject(s): _____

Range of Motion Measurements		
Body part used	**Pre-Application**	**Post-Application**

▊ Activity Questions

1. Paraffin is heated to a temperature of around 120°F, a water temperature that would be intolerable for therapeutic purposes. Why is the temperature of paraffin therapeutic and not harmful?

2. Based on the make-up of a paraffin bath, what are some special precautions you should be aware of when treating athletes, general public, or elderly patients?

3. What is the purpose of dipping the extremity 6 to 12 times?

On completion of the activities for Unit 2, review the following case studies to enhance practical application of superficial heat modalities.

1. A 33-year-old secretary has just been released to begin rehabilitation after a fracture/dislocation to the PIP joint of the index finger from a fall. You notice a decrease in PIP ROM. What modality would you begin with and why?

2. You have a football player who sustained a turf toe injury during last Friday's game. It is now Wednesday, and ROM is still lacking. You determine that a heat modality is indicated. What modality would you use and why?

Other Thermal Agents

Background and Discussion

Thermal agents are often used to facilitate soft-tissue flexibility and joint range of motion (ROM). The reasons for choosing cold or heat therapy range from the stage of the injury being treated to the preference of the individual being treated. Cold may be preferred because of its pain-reducing capacity; heat may be selected for its effects on collagen extensibility. Regardless of the choice, the clinician must remember that the modality is only as effective as the therapeutic exercise subsequently used.

Hydrotherapy, when used properly, is a safe treatment modality. Water has a relatively high specific heat and thermal conductivity. Thus, the use of whirlpools for the treatment of orthopaedic injuries has been supported in the literature. The temperature of the water for either hot or cold treatments is dependent on the proportion of the body immersed. Contrast therapy is the alternating of hot and cold modalities during a treatment session. The time ratio for alternating between hot and cold is variable (e.g., 3:1 for 3 minutes of cold and 1 minute of hot). Physiological benefits of contrast treatments have been questioned in the literature. Theoretically, the change from hot to cold is thought to create a "pumping-type" action to enhance circulation for the reduction of edema.

However, most treatment parameters do not allow for a large enough temperature gradient between the hot and cold phases to result in physiological benefits.

Contraindications

- Please refer to Units 1 and 2 for a listing of contraindications to cold and heat modalities.
  Additional contraindications specific to hydrotherapy (including full or nearly full immersion):
- Acute conditions when turbulence of the water in a whirlpool would irritate the condition
- Cardiac instability
- Fever (hot whirlpool)
- Severe respiratory conditions
- Poor thermal regulation
- Infectious conditions capable of being spread through water
- Severe epilepsy
- Urinary/bowel incontinence
- Pregnancy (in very warm water)
- Fear of water
- Limited strength or balance (precaution)

Effect of Heat, Cold, and Static Stretch on Tissue Elasticity

Objective

To determine the effects of heat and cold application and stretching on tissue elasticity and joint ROM.

Materials Needed

- Ice pack
- Moist heat pack
- Goniometer
- Measurement of hamstring flexibility

Several methods may be used to determine the flexibility of the hamstring group, including sit-and-reach, stand-and-reach, and goniometric measurements of hip flexion with the knee extended. For the purposes of this exercise, the method used must be objective so that the pre-test and post-test scores can be measured accurately. We recommend the use of goniometric measurements, although any objective method may be used.

To measure hip flexion, begin with the subject lying supine. Align the stationary arm along the subject's torso so that it remains parallel with the tabletop, align the axis with the greater trochanter, and align the moveable arm with the femoral shaft, using the lateral epicondyle as a landmark. The hip is then flexed to its maximal ROM (Fig. 3–1). To avoid a false representation of available hip motion, ensure that lumbopelvic motion does not occur.

Hamstring Stretching

Hamstring stretching can take many forms. For this exercise, a modified hurdler's stretch is recommended (Fig. 3–2). Avoiding lumbar flexion, subjects should move into the

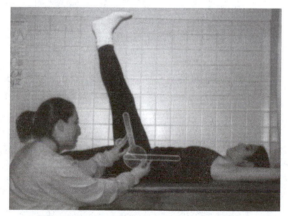

Figure 3–1.   Measurement of hip ROM.

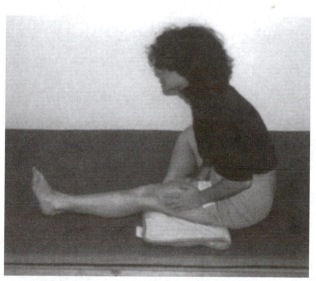

Figure 3–2.   Modified hurdler's stretch.

stretch and maintain the position where a comfortable tightness is noted.

Procedures

1. Select one of the following five treatments if your instructor has not assigned one to you.
   - Heat only
   - Heat with concurrent stretch
   - Ice only
   - Ice with concurrent stretch
   - Stretch only
   For smaller classes, students can do a different condition on each leg.
2. Determine the baseline amount of hamstring flexibility, and record it on the worksheet.
3. Apply the modality (hot or cold) to both hamstring groups, using the proper protocol for 10 minutes.

Those who are assigned to stretch should perform a modified hurdler's stretch (30 seconds on; 30 seconds off) during the treatment.

4. Immediately after the treatment is over, remove the modality, remeasure the amount of hamstring flexibility, and record it on the worksheet.
5. Calculate the net increase or decrease in the ROM.
6. Using the values obtained by the class; categorize the pre-test and post-test scores using the chart provided.
7. Statistical analysis, such as the t-Test, may be used to determine if there is a significant difference between the techniques.

Note

For the heat-plus-stretch combination, use adequate toweling, and advise the subject to add more toweling or discontinue the exercise if the hot pack becomes too warm.

Effect of Heat, Cold, and Static Stretch on Tissue Elasticity

Name: _____   Date: _____

Subject(s): _____

Subject	Modality Used	Pre-Test ROM	Post-Test ROM
#1	☐ Heat ☐ Cold ☐ Stretch		
#2	☐ Heat ☐ Cold ☐ Stretch		
#3	☐ Heat ☐ Cold ☐ Stretch		
#4	☐ Heat ☐ Cold ☐ Stretch		
#5	☐ Heat ☐ Cold ☐ Stretch		
#6	☐ Heat ☐ Cold ☐ Stretch		
#7	☐ Heat ☐ Cold ☐ Stretch		
#8	☐ Heat ☐ Cold ☐ Stretch		

Cold Application			
Subject	Pre	Post	Difference

Heat Application			
Subject	Pre	Post	Difference

Cold & Stretch Application			
Subject	Pre	Post	Difference

Heat & Stretch Application			
Subject	Pre	Post	Difference

Activity Questions

1. Using the information obtained from all subjects, which treatment condition resulted in the greatest increase in hamstring flexibility? How could you clinically apply this information in treating a patient with limited hamstring flexibility?

2. Compare the changes in hamstring flexibility between conditions using a modality alone, those using a modality plus concurrent stretching, and stretching alone. Hypothesize your findings if you were to take hamstring measurements tomorrow.

Contrast Therapy: Skin Temperature Changes

Objective

To determine the relative effectiveness of contrast therapy in changing the skin surface temperature.

Materials Needed

- Surface temperature gauge
- Timing device
- Various methods of delivering heat and cold:
  - Moist heat pack
  - Warm whirlpool (WWP)/warm water immersion
  - Ice bag
  - Cold whirlpool (CWP)/cold water immersion

Procedures

1. Be sure the patient is free from contraindications relative to the modalities that will be used during this activity.
2. Using the surface temperature gauge, record the baseline skin temperature of the area to be treated. Record this reading on the chart provided.
3. Apply the heat modality to the body part in the prescribed manner for a total of 3 minutes. Record the skin temperature at the end of the 3 minutes.
4. Apply the cold modality to the body part in the prescribed manner for a total of 1 minute. Record the skin temperature at the end of the minute.

   OPTIONAL: If an electronic skin temperature probe is available and the particular modality makes it feasible, measure the changes in skin temperature during the heat and cold applications, and recorded the findings in the 3:1 minute intervals. Insulate the side of the probe exposed to the modalities to limit influence from the modality itself. Failure to insulate the probe may result in temperature recording that reflects the temperature of the skin-modality interface.
5. Repeat Procedures 3 and 4 three additional times. Remeasure the skin temperature every time there is a change between the hot and cold (modality).
6. On completion of four cycles of contrast treatment, begin recording the skin temperature every 2 minutes until the temperature returns to the baseline value or the 20-minute post-treatment period has expired.
7. On completion of the activity, plot the changes in skin temperature resulting from each modality. Students are encouraged to enter data into a spreadsheet and plot it to view the temperature changes graphically.

Note: If using warm and cold whirlpools for the contrast therapy, the temperatures should be between 105°F and 110°F (40.6°C to 43.3°C) for the WWP and 50°F and 60°F (10°C to 15.6°C) for the CWP.

Contrast Therapy: Skin Temperature Changes

Name: _____   Date: _____

Subject(s): _____

Modalities used _____

	Baseline	Contrast Treatment								
	0	3	4	7	8	11	12	15	16
Skin temperature									

	Baseline	Post-Application										
	0	2	4	6	8	10	12	14	16	18	20
Skin temperature											

On graph paper or a spreadsheet program, plot the changes in skin temperature that occurred during the contrast therapy treatment. Use this graph to answer the Activity Questions.

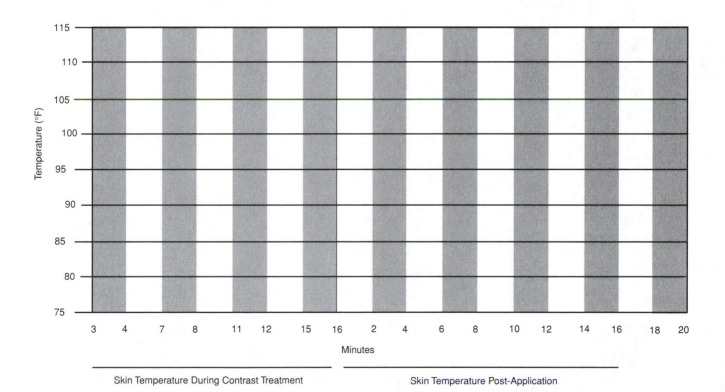

Activity Questions

1. What was greatest skin temperature increase? What was the greatest skin temperature decrease?

2. Compare the findings of the skin temperature increases and decreases in this activity with those of Activities 1–1 and 2–1. Which condition demonstrated the longer time for return to normal skin temperature?

3. Do you think there was a sufficient change in temperature to promote physiological changes superficially? Is your answer the same for deep tissues?

After competing the activities for Unit 3, review the following case studies to enhance practical application of superficial heat modalities.

1. The local school's best singles tennis player has just suffered a grade 1 hamstring strain, and it is 7 days before the conference match. Using the information provided, how will you treat this injury? Her signs and symptoms are:
   a. Pain: 4/10
   b. Nearly full AROM
   c. Manual muscle test:
      Knee flexion: 4/5
      Knee extension: 5/5
      Hip extension: 4+/5
   d. Slight swelling

2. A 29-year-old man comes to you for help on a Monday after competing in a weekend power-lifting competition. He is complaining of soreness in his biceps bilaterally (5/10) and has decreased elbow extension. There is no indication of significant trauma, and the injury appears to be associated with delayed onset of muscle soreness. He is a construction worker and needs to be able to return to work quickly. How would you treat this patient?

Electrical Stimulation Modalities

Background and Discussion

The use of electrical stimulation incorporates a wide variety of application techniques. Electrical stimulators are becoming increasingly sophisticated, with single machines frequently capable of generating several currents. Many find this intimidating; however, the fundamentals remain the same. Knowledge of these fundamentals enables the practitioner to become familiar quickly with the capabilities of any unit (regardless of how it is packaged) and underscores the fact that a single current type can be manipulated to provide a wide range of effects. One patient's perceptions of the relative comfort of a specific parameter may differ dramatically from those of another patient. Some parameters (e.g., frequency) must be set in a specified range to achieve a specific therapeutic effect. Other parameters (e.g., shape of the wave) can be adjusted according to personal preference without negatively influencing desired treatment effects.[12]

Some protocols call for sensory-level stimulation only, whereas others use an electrically induced muscle contraction. Occasionally, even a noxious (painful) stimulus is desired. Each of these sensations results from the response of a particular type of nerve. Whether a nerve fires in response to electrical stimulation is determined by the nerve's diameter and depth and by the pulse duration and intensity of the stimulation.

The larger the diameter of the nerve, the lower its resistance and the lower the amplitude necessary for its stimulation. Logically, deeper nerves require a greater amplitude for stimulation than more superficial nerves. In normal, innervated tissue, the order in which nerves are stimulated is constant. As the intensity is increased, sensory fibers are stimulated first, followed by motor nerves and then pain fibers. If the intensity is increased past the point of pain, muscle fibers are then directly stimulated. Short pulse durations allow for the greatest selectivity in the stimulation of these fibers. As the pulse duration is increased, the amount of selectivity between the individual fibers is decreased.

An electrical current travels through the body by forming a sequence of parallel circuits, opting for the path of least resistance. Changing the configuration of the electrode placement alters the path of the current, although the area of greatest current density remains directly under the electrode(s) with the smallest surface area. Little or no stimulation is detected under the dispersive electrode when a monopolar configuration is used because the surface area of the dispersive electrode is greater than the surface area of the treatment pads. The depth of the treatment effect corresponds to the proximity of the electrodes, with the depth increasing as the space between the electrodes increases. When the subject shifts off the dispersive electrode during treatment or the conducting medium dries out, a greater current density occurs along this diminished pathway. The perceived sensation increases, sometimes painfully so. For this reason, gel or gel-impregnated electrodes are often used as a coupling agent instead of water when electrical stimulation is applied over a long period. The gels are less apt to dry out and therefore deliver current at a constant density.

The DC generator (e.g., Iontophoresor) creates a continuous electromotive field between the anode and cathode. This allows for migration of hydrogen toward the cathode and oxygen to the anode. These lines of force between the poles of a monophasic generator are less distinct because of the interruption in the current flow. During the periods of noncurrent flow, the ions are capable of drifting freely in any direction, ultimately reducing the net migration of the ions. Direct evidence of the effects of stimulation using a galvanic current occurs when burns result from build-up of acid or alkaline by-products.[16] Because of this risk, only low amplitude and short durations are used with this current type. Decreasing skin impedance through procedures such as shaving and warming also helps reduce these undesirable side effects.

When using electrical stimulation to elicit a muscular contraction, the placement of the electrodes greatly influences the amount of current necessary to elicit a contraction. Placing the electrodes directly over motor points produces a maximum motor response using a minimum of current. If the current density over the muscle or muscle group is kept high, more motor points (and therefore motor units) will be recruited into the contraction. Increasing the output intensity by stimulating motor nerves in adjacent areas also has the same effect.

In theory, the polarity used (when a choice is possible) can also affect the motor response. According to Pflueger's law, less current is required to depolarize a nerve at the cathode (negative pole) than at the anode.[13] Of course, this is only meaningful when a direct or monophasic current is used.

Motor points, however, are not the only areas of decreased electrical resistance. Acupuncture points and trigger points also demonstrate diminished surface electrical resistance. Located on meridians, acupuncture points, theoretically, are entrances into different energy systems of the body. Trigger points, motor points, and acupuncture points are often painful to palpation in the presence of injury.

Almost any type of electrotherapeutic modality can elicit a muscle contraction in normal, healthy muscle. All that is needed is sufficient intensity to depolarize the motor nerve's membrane. Certain forms of electrical stimulation may depolarize the motor nerve's membrane more easily and with greater comfort. While electrical stimulation is capable of producing involuntary muscle contractions, combining electrical stimulation with volitional muscle contraction can produce contractions that exceed the maximal voluntary isometric contraction.

It should be noted that the overall strength of a muscle is affected more through voluntary muscle contractions than through electrically induced muscle contractions. Electrical stimulation produces less desirable muscle contractions than voluntary contractions but can be used to supplement and augment voluntary contractions. This should drive the clinician to use electrical stimulation not as a replacement for voluntary contractions but as a supplement to voluntary contractions.

When using electrically induced muscle contractions for strength gains, the effect of fatigue must be considered. As with all exercises and muscle contractions, a rest time is needed to allow the muscles to recuperate. Treatment sessions with electrically induced muscle contractions should occur every other day as is typical of normal workouts. Increasing strength is most effective when recruiting the maximal number of muscle fibers. This should be kept in mind when choosing pulse frequencies. Lower frequencies result in twitch contractions, which do not recruit the largest amount of muscle fibers. Higher frequencies result in tetanic or tonic muscle contractions, which recruit larger numbers of muscle fibers.

The types of muscle fibers that are recruited in electrically induced muscle contractions must be kept in mind. Electrical stimulation reverses the order of recruitment of muscle fibers. In voluntary contractions, small-diameter type I motor nerves are first to be recruited. In electrically induced muscle contractions, type II motor nerves are first to be recruited. Type II motor nerves are capable of producing more force but also fatigue quickly, whereas type I fibers are able to sustain lower force contractions for prolonged periods.

Cold application has been thought to decrease pain by decreasing the excitability of the pain-causing free nerve endings, stimulating large-diameter neurons, "closing the gate" as described by the gate control theory, and evoking descending inhibition through the central biasing mechanism. Cold modalities are frequently used for a temporary reduction of pain to enhance the subsequent treatment. For example, cold might be used before or during potentially painful active range-of-motion exercises in a technique known as cryokinetics. Additionally, pain caused by the stimulating current determines the upper limits of torque production.

Research studies have been conducted to determine if cold application prior to electrical stimulation alters the torque produced by an electrically evoked muscle contraction. One study using ice massage as the method for delivering cold found a significant increase in torque production among subjects receiving such treatment compared with those receiving no such treatment.[14] A similar study using ice bags found no significant difference between the two groups.[15]

■ Contraindications

General
- Cardiac disability
- Exposed metal implants, such as those used for external fixation
- Severe obesity
- Over areas of particular sensitivity
- Carotid sinus
- Esophagus (laryngeal or pharyngeal muscles)
- Pharynx
- Mucosal membranes
- During pregnancy
- Skin irritation due to electrode placement

Motor-Level Stimulation
- Unwanted muscle contraction or active movement
- Hemorrhage or active inflammation
- Malignancies

Direct Current (Iontophoresis)
- Anesthetic skin
- Recent scars
- Metal implants
- Exposed metal
- Acute injury
- Cardiac pacemakers
- Contraindications or sensitivity to the medication(s) being used

Ohm's Law

■ Objective

To demonstrate an understanding of the relationship between voltage, amperage, resistance, and the power of an electrical circuit.

■ Description of Ohm's Law

Ohm's law is a mathematical equation that describes a relationship in which amperage (I) is directly proportional to voltage (V) and inversely proportional to resistance (R). Expressed as an equation, each variable can be calculated if the other two variables are known. To calculate:

Amperage	Voltage	Resistance
$I = V/R$	$V = IR$	$R = V/I$

The total resistance to current flow is based on the type of electrical circuit involved. In a series circuit where the electrons have only one path to travel, the total resistance is equal to the sum of all the resistors:

$$R_t = r_1 + r_2 + r_3 \dots$$

In a parallel circuit, where electrons have multiple routes to travel, the total resistance is inversely proportional to the sum of the individual resistors:

$$1/R_t = 1/r_1 + 1/r_2 + 1/r_3$$

The power of a circuit is described in terms of watts and is calculated by the equation:

$$P = VI$$

■ Definition of Terms

Amperage (I):   The rate of electrical current flow as measured by the number of coulombs passing a single point in 1 second. 1 ampere is equal to the movement of one coulomb per second.

Coulomb (Q):   Charge produced by 6.25×10^{18} electrons.

Ohm (Ω):   Unit of electrical resistance. 1 ohm is the amount of resistance needed to develop 0.24 calories of heat when 1 ampere of current is applied for 1 second.

Voltage (V):   The potential for electron flow to occur. 1 volt represents the amount of work required to move 1 coulomb of charge.

Watt (W):   Unit of electrical power that describes the amount of work being performed in a unit of time.

Ohm's Law

Name: _____   Date: _____

Respond to the following questions using the schematics provided below. Show your work.

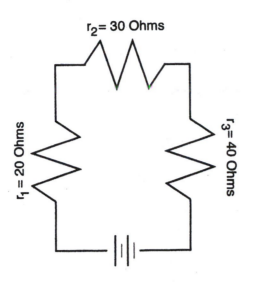

Series Circuit   **Parallel Circuit**

1. What is the total resistance in the series circuit? The parallel circuit?

2. Using the resistance value obtained in Question 1, what would be the amperage of each circuit if each is operating at 120 volts?

3. What would the amperage for each of the two circuits be if the voltage were increased to 200 volts?

4. Using the parameters from Question 2, what would the wattage be for each circuit type?

5. Calculate the voltage across each resistor in the series circuit, assuming the circuit is operating at 10 amperes.

6. Calculate the amperage across each resistor in the parallel circuit, assuming it is operating at 100 volts and 10 amperes.

7. Calculate the total resistance in the parallel circuit after adding two additional resistors of 30 ohms each.

8. Using the total resistance value obtained from Question 7, calculate the amperage if the circuit is operating at 120 volts.

9. Compare your answers to Questions 8 and 2 for the amperage of the parallel circuit. After adding resistance, did the amperage increase or decrease? Why?

Selective Stimulation of Nerves

Objective

To understand how adjustment of the pulse duration affects the level of intensity required to stimulate sensory, motor, and pain nerve fibers.

Materials Needed

- Electrical stimulation unit with an adjustable pulse duration (TENS or neuromuscular electrical stimulation recommended). Units with a digital output display produce the most objective results.

Procedures

1. Depending on the stimulating unit used, select either a monopolar or bipolar electrode configuration. When using a monopolar electrode configuration, attach the "dispersive" electrode on the subject's lower back or thigh and the "active" electrode to the anterior portion of the subject's forearm. (This configuration is recommended for high-volt pulsed units). If other stimulators are used, arrange the electrodes in a bipolar configuration, placing one electrode on the distal portion of the subject's forearm and the other on the proximal portion of the forearm (Fig. 4–1).
2. Set the stimulation parameters to the following values:

Parameters	Settings
Pulse duration:	25 μsec (or lowest possible value)
Pulse frequency:	30 pps
Pad alternating rate:	Continuous
Modulation parameters:	Off (constant output)
Duty cycle:	100%
Polarity:	Positive

   Note: Not all parameters will apply to each unit.
3. Position the stimulation unit so that the subject cannot see the intensity reading.
4. Slowly increase the intensity to the level where the subject first reports the sensation of electrical current flow. Record the output intensity on the grid provided.
5. Further increase the intensity until a visible muscle contraction can be seen, and record the output intensity.
6. Continue to increase the intensity until the subject reports discomfort resulting from the stimulation. Reduce the intensity to zero, and record the output intensity
7. Allow the subject recovery time from the stimulation bout.
8. Repeat Steps 3 through 7 using increased pulse durations (e.g., 10 μsec, 20 μsec, 40 μsec, 80 μsec, and 160 μsec).
9. Conclude this activity using the original pulse duration.
10. Using the labeling key provided, plot the changes in the output intensity required to stimulate sensory nerves, motor nerves, and pain nerves between the various pulse durations.

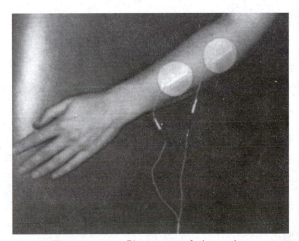

Figure 4–1. Placement of electrodes.

Selective Stimulation of Nerves

Name: _____   Date: _____

Subject(s): _____

Type of Stimulation Unit Used: _____

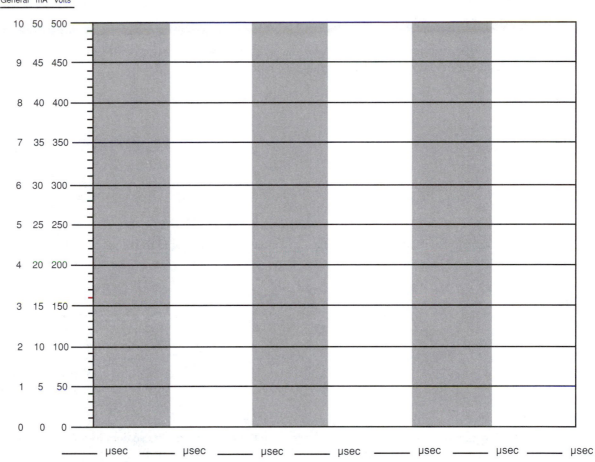

Metered Output

General   mA   Volts

10	50	500
9	45	450
8	40	400
7	35	350
6	30	300
5	25	250
4	20	200
3	15	150
2	10	100
1	5	50
0	0	0

_____ μsec   _____ μsec   _____ μsec   _____ μsec   _____ μsec   _____ μsec   _____ μsec

Pulse Duration

Labeling Key

○ Sensory Nerves   ☐ Pain Nerves

● Motor Nerves

■ Activity Questions

1. Was the interval between sensory, motor, and pain stimulation reduced as the pulse duration was increased? Based on these results, what can you infer about the comfort level of an uninterrupted direct current (galvanic)?

2. Based on your results, what would be the optimal pulse duration if your treatment goal was to achieve maximal sensory stimulation without muscle contraction?

3. Note that the electrode-skin interface will affect resistance. Does the actual amplitude reading have any clinical relevance? Why or why not?

4. Compare the two first and last readings using the same shortest pulse duration. Were they the same? To what do you attribute any difference?

Pulse Characteristics

Objective

To demonstrate knowledge of the characteristics associated with therapeutic currents.

Electrical Stimulating Currents

Direct Current: The uninterrupted unidirectional flow of electrons.

Alternating Current: The uninterrupted bidirectional flow of electrons.

Pulsed Current: The flow of electrons interrupted by discrete periods of noncurrent flow.

Monophasic Current: A unidirectional pulsed current.

Biphasic Current: A pulsed current possessing two phases, each of which occurs on opposite sides of the baseline.

Definition of Pulse Characteristics

Amplitude: The maximal distance that a pulse rises above or below the baseline.

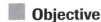

Interpulse Interval: The period of time between pulses during which there is no current flow.

Intrapulse Interval: The period of time within a single pulse during which there is no current flow. The duration of the intrapulse interval cannot exceed the duration of the interpulse interval.

Peak-to-Peak Amplitude: The absolute value measured from the maximal rise on the positive side of the baseline to the peak on the negative side.

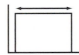

Pulse Duration: The period of time a pulse remains above or below the baseline, normally measured in microseconds.

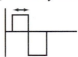

Phase Duration: The period of time a phase remains above or below the baseline, normally measured in microseconds.

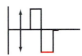

Pulse Frequency: With pulsed currents, this figure represents the number of pulses per second (pps); alternating currents are measured by the number of cycles per second (cps or hertz).

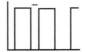

One Second

Pulse Period: The period of time between the initiation of one pulse to the initiation of the subsequent pulse.

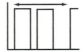

Pulse Characteristics

Name: _____   Date: _____

1. Label each of the following current types, indicating the specified parameter. If a particular parameter is not applicable to a particular current, leave it blank.
   A. Identify the amplitude for each of the following currents:

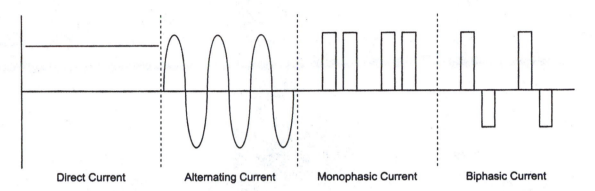

| Direct Current | Alternating Current | Monophasic Current | Biphasic Current |

B. Identify the peak-to-peak value for each of the following currents:

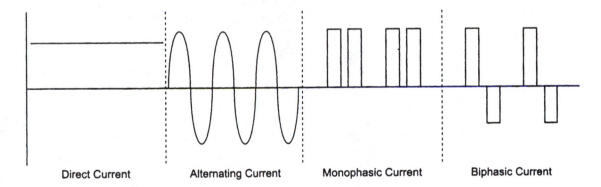

| Direct Current | Alternating Current | Monophasic Current | Biphasic Current |

C. Identify the pulse duration for each of the following currents:

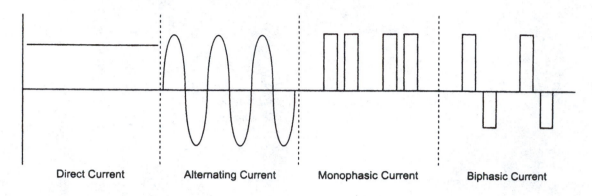

| Direct Current | Alternating Current | Monophasic Current | Biphasic Current |

D. Identify the phase duration for each of the following currents:

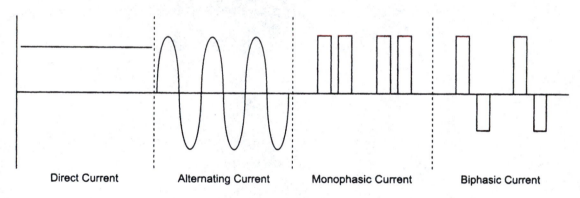

| Direct Current | Alternating Current | Monophasic Current | Biphasic Current |

E. Identify the pulse period for each of the following currents:

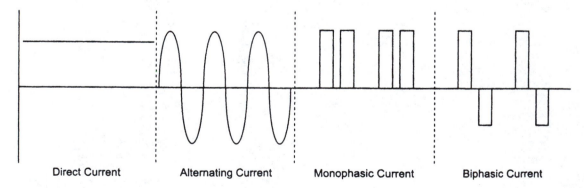

| Direct Current | Alternating Current | Monophasic Current | Biphasic Current |

F. Identify the interpulse interval for each of the following currents:

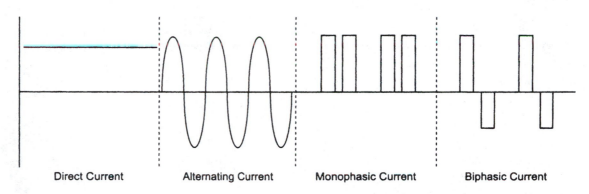

Direct Current   Alternating Current   Monophasic Current   Biphasic Current

G. Identify the intrapulse interval for each of the following currents.

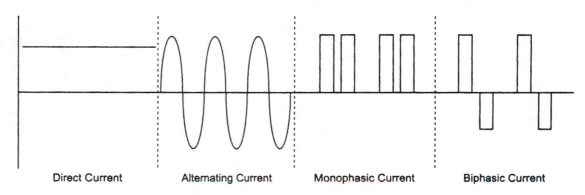

Direct Current   Alternating Current   Monophasic Current   Biphasic Current

2. Calculate the total amount of time electrons are actually moving during a 1-minute period in a pulsed current having a pulse duration of 140 μsec and a frequency of 125 pps. Show your work.

3. The amount of energy delivered to the tissue is represented by the area within a pulse. What two variables can we manipulate to increase or decrease this energy?

Current Density

Objective

To understand the effects of current density on the perception of electrical current flow.

Materials Needed

- Immersion bucket (filled at least 11 inches deep with warm water)
- Electrical stimulation (ES) unit designed to operate when the electrodes are submerged in water (high-volt pulsed stimulation recommended)

Description of Concurrent Immersion and Electrical Stimulation

Electrical stimulation may be delivered to a large area by immersing the body part in a tub of water (during therapeutic treatments, the temperature of the water is cold for acute injuries and warm/hot for more chronic conditions). One lead, usually a "dispersive" electrode, is attached to the subject while the active electrode is immersed in the water (Fig. 4–2). In this configuration, the water touching the immersed extremity (through its length, around its circumference, and around the length and circumference of the phalanges) serves as an interface for conducting the current.

The patient's perception of an electrical current is based on two factors: the intensity of the output and the density of the current under the electrode. Consider a current of 300 volts flowing through an electrode of 10 square inches: the resultant current density would be 30 volts per square inch. If the size of the electrode were reduced to 5 square inches, the current density would be 60 volts per square inch. Assuming that the intensity of the output remains the same, the perception of the stimulus would be greater with the smaller electrodes than with the larger electrodes.

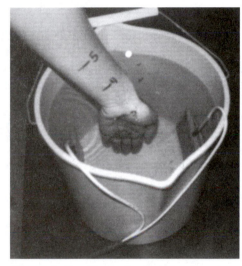

Figure 4–2.   Electrodes immerse in water.

Procedure

IT IS IMPORTANT THAT THE SUBJECT DOES NOT COMPLETELY REMOVE THE HAND FROM THE WATER WHILE THE CURRENT IS FLOWING! Please advise your subject of this caveat before proceeding, and provide regular reminders throughout this exercise.

- If the stimulator is operated by standard current, ensure that it is plugged into a ground fault interrupter.
  1. On the subject's nondominant anterior hand and forearm, measure 2 inches proximally from the tip of the middle finger, and make a transverse mark. Label this mark "1." Moving proximally in 2-inch increments, mark and label lines "2" through "5" (Fig. 4–3).
  2. Place one or two electrodes in the tub of water, and position them so that the rubber insulating material is

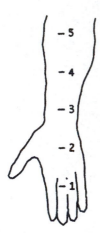

Figure 4–3.   Hand and arm markings.

facing inward toward the center of the bucket (see Fig. 4–2).

3. Instruct the subject not to touch the electrodes or the stimulation unit at any time during this exercise.

4. With the subject seated, fasten a large dispersive electrode to the subject's thigh on the same side as the active electrode. The subject's arm will be immersed in the water in a later step.

5. Set the stimulation parameters to the following values:

Parameters	Settings
Pulse duration:	25 to 50 μsec
Pulse frequency:	100 pps
Pad alternating rate:	Continuous
Modulation parameters:	Off (constant output)
Duty cycle:	100%

Note: Not all parameters will apply to each unit.

6. Make sure that the output intensity is reduced to zero.

7. Instruct the subject to immerse the arm in the water to the "5" mark. For safety, remind the subject again not to completely remove the arm from the water while the current is flowing. Instruct the subject to re-immerse the arm, not withdraw it, if the intensity becomes too great.

8. Slowly increase the intensity to the level at which the subject first experiences the sensation of an electrical current. Using the Numerical Rating Scale, have the subject record the perceived intensity of the stimulus. Cover this and future responses to prevent them from influencing the subject's subsequent ratings.

9. Instruct the subject to gradually withdraw the arm to the "4" mark, and record the perceived intensity of the stimulus.

10. Repeat the same sequence so that the subject moves to the "3," "2," and "1" mark, and record the perceived stimulus for each. Note that some subjects will not be able to tolerate the stimulus at the "2" or "1" level. If this is case, have the subject record the perception of the tolerable stimulus, reduce the intensity to zero, and conclude the activity.

Current Density

Name: _____ Date: _____

Subject(s): _____

Type of Stimulation Unit Used: _____

Stimulus Perception at the Level "5" Mark

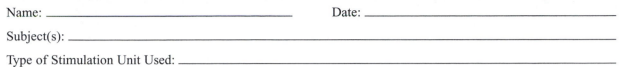

Stimulus Perception at the Level "4" Mark

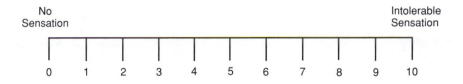

Stimulus Perception at the Level "3" Mark

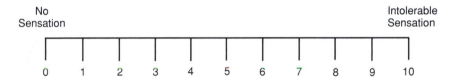

Stimulus Perception at the Level "2" Mark

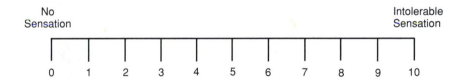

Stimulus Perception at the Level "1" Mark

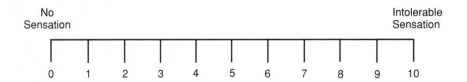

Activity Questions:

1. It was emphasized that the subject should not completely remove the arm from the immersion bucket while the current was flowing. Why should this be avoided?

2. When performing testing for this laboratory exercise, some students report perception decreases as the limb is slowly removed? What explanation might you provide for this result?

3. As you are increasing the current intensity during an ES treatment with a monopolar electrode arrangement, the person describes feeling the current primarily at the dispersive electrode. Identify at least three steps you could take to have stimulation perceived under the active electrode only.

Identification of Motor Points

■ Objective

To be able to locate and identify motor points for specific muscles.

■ Materials Needed

- Electrical stimulation unit with a hand-held applicator (high-volt pulsed stimulator recommended)

■ Description of Motor Points

Motor points are superficial areas on the skin that have decreased resistance to electrical current flow. Stimulation of these sites causes large motor nerves to depolarize and therefore isolates the contraction to a single muscle or portion of a muscle. The exact locations of motor points tend to vary from individual to individual, but their approximate locations have been identified in many motor point charts. Motor points are not to be confused with trigger points, which are hypersensitive areas that develop secondary to trauma (although they do frequently tend to be found close to each other).

■ Procedures

1. Attach the dispersive electrode to the subject's thigh or upper arm, depending on the area being examined, and configure the stimulation unit to the hand-held applicator mode. On units not having a provision for a hand-held probe, a small (e.g., 2-inch × 2-inch) electrode can be used. In this case, attach the dispersive electrode to the subject's thigh or upper arm, and manually move the electrode with one hand while controlling the output intensity with the other.

2. Set the stimulation parameters to the following values:

Parameters	Settings
Pulse duration:	25 to 50 μsec
Pulse frequency:	50 pps
Pad alternating rate:	Continuous
Modulation parameters:	Off (constant output)
Polarity of the active electrode:	Negative
Duty cycle:	100%

Note: Not all parameters will apply to each unit.

3. Reset the generator's output intensity to zero, and wet the applicator's tip with water or gel.

4. Place the applicator tip on the subject's forearm, and slowly increase the intensity to where a slight muscle contraction is visible (Fig. 4–4).

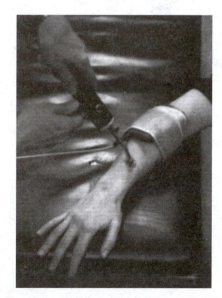

Figure 4–4. Use of hand-held applicator.

5. Use the applicator tip to identify the point(s) on the skin that result in strong, isolated contractions of the following muscles:

Upper Extremity	*Lower Extremity*
Abductor pollicis longus	Abductor digiti minimi
Extensor digiti minimi	Extensor hallucis longus
Extensor indicis	Extensor digitorum brevis
Flexor carpi radialis	Plantaris
Flexor carpi ulnaris	Tibialis anterior

6. The intensity of the stimulation may need to be adjusted as the applicator is moved over the skin. Most applicators have an intensity adjustment knob located on them. *Note:* Reduce the intensity to zero before applying or removing the applicator from the subject's skin.

7. Using the labeling key, mark the location of each motor point identified on the accompanying charts.

Identification of Motor Points

Name: _____   Date: _____

Subject(s): _____

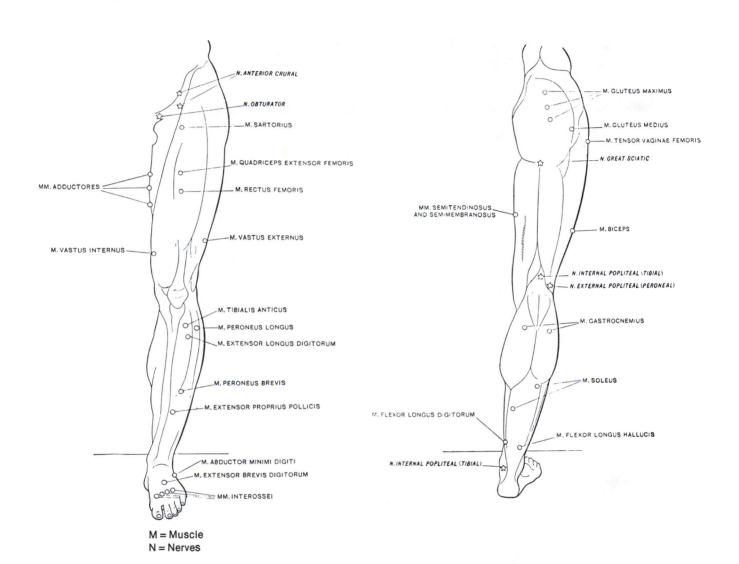

M = Muscle
N = Nerves

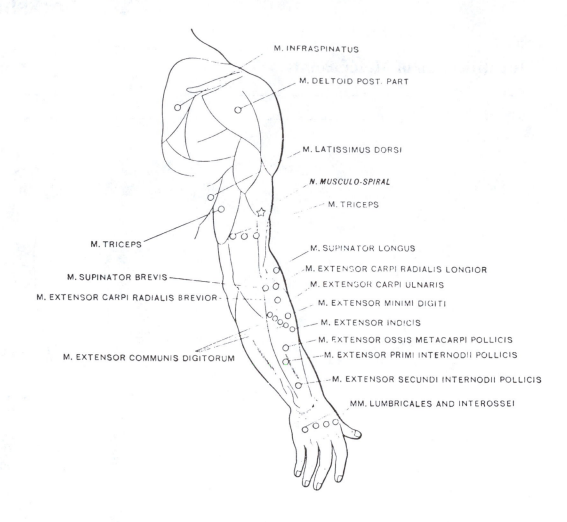

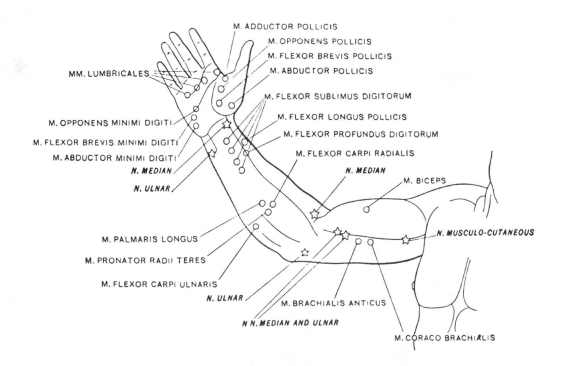

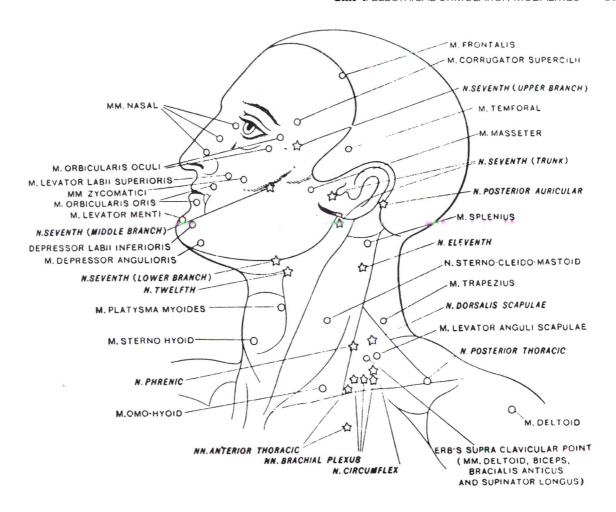

MM. NASAL

M. FRONTALIS

M. CORRUGATOR SUPERCILII

N. SEVENTH (UPPER BRANCH)

M. TEMFORAL

M. MASSETER

N. SEVENTH (TRUNK)

N. POSTERIOR AURICULAR

M. ORBICULARIS OCULI

M. LEVATOR LABII SUPERIORIS

MM. ZYCOMATICI

M. ORBICULARIS ORIS

M. LEVATOR MENTI

N. SEVENTH (MIDDLE BRANCH)

DEPRESSOR LABII INFERIORIS

M. DEPRESSOR ANGULIORIS

N. SEVENTH (LOWER BRANCH)

N. TWELFTH

M. PLATYSMA MYOIDES

M. STERNO HYOID

N. PHRENIC

M. OMO-HYOID

M. SPLENIUS

N. ELEVENTH

N. STERNO-CLEIDO-MASTOID

M. TRAPEZIUS

N. DORSALIS SCAPULAE

M. LEVATOR ANGULI SCAPULAE

N. POSTERIOR THORACIC

M. DELTOID

ERB'S SUPRA CLAVICULAR POINT
(MM. DELTOID, BICEPS,
BRACIALIS ANTICUS
AND SUPINATOR LONGUS)

NN. ANTERIOR THORACIC

NN. BRACHIAL PLEXUS

N. CIRCUMFLEX

Labeling Key

Upper Extremity
 1. Abductor pollicis longus
 2. Extensor digiti minimi
 3. Extensor indicis
 4. Flexor carpi radialis
 5. Flexor carpi ulnaris
 6. Other:
 7. Other:
 8. Other:
 9. Other:
10. Other:

Lower Extremity
A. Abductor digiti minima
B. Extensor hallicus longus
C. Peroneus longus
D. Extensor digitorum brevis
E. Tibialis anterior
 F. Other:
G. Other:
H. Other:
 I. Other:
 J. Other:

▨ Activity Questions

 1. Compare your findings with those of your subject. Do the motor points approximate those on the chart? What would explain any differences?

2. If you are using a unit where a polarity change is possible, try the following: Change the polarity from negative to positive. Move to an identified motor point and increase the intensity until a similar contraction is elicited. Did the required intensity change from your initial trial?

3. Is it possible to obtain a muscle contraction if electrode placement is not over a motor point? Why or why not?

Manual Determination of Optimal Stimulation Sites

Objective

To manually determine superficial points on the skin having a decreased resistance to electrical stimulation, indicating primary stimulation points.

Materials Needed

- Transcutaneous electrical nerve stimulation (TENS) unit or other electrical stimulator capable of a bipolar arrangement.

Procedures

1. Using one channel of the TENS unit, set the stimulation parameters to the following values:

Parameters	Settings
Pulse duration:	20 μsec
Pulse frequency:	120 pps
Modulation parameters:	Off (constant output)

2. If required, apply conductive gel to each electrode. Attach one electrode to your dominant forearm and attach the other electrode to the subject's upper arm or lower leg, depending on the area being examined.
3. Apply a dab of conductive gel to the index finger of your dominant hand.
4. Touch the subject's extremity being examined (e.g., the forearm).
5. Slowly increase the output intensity of the TENS unit until a slight sensation is felt under your finger.
6. Slowly move your finger over the body area, and note locations of increased sensation and whether or not a muscle contraction is associated with the particular point (Fig. 4–5). Label these locations on the chart provided.
7. Repeat this activity using another body part (e.g., the lower leg).

Notes

1. If the electrical stimulator being used is equipped with an ohm meter, this exercise can be used to compare perceived sensations with the output of the ohm meter.
2. Ohm meters are often incorporated into many point stimulators to locate these optimal stimulation sites exactly. As with motor points, the locations of these sites can be approximated using charts. In this activity, your finger serves as a quasi–ohm meter, and rather than a metered output to measure the amount of current flow, you are relying on your perception of the stimulus.

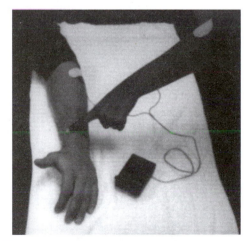

Figure 4–5. Manual location of stimulation site.

Manual Determination of Optimal Stimulation Sites

Name: _____   Date: _____

Subject(s): _____

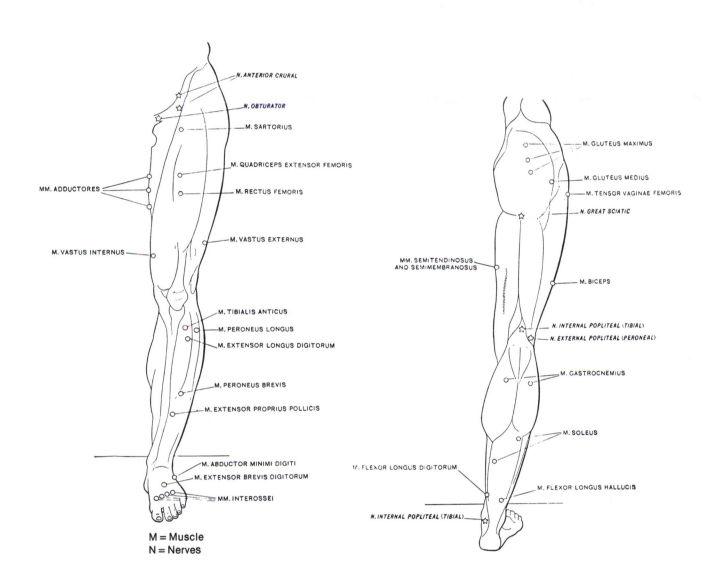

N. ANTERIOR CRURAL

N. OBTURATOR

M. SARTORIUS

M. QUADRICEPS EXTENSOR FEMORIS

MM. ADDUCTORES

M. RECTUS FEMORIS

M. VASTUS EXTERNUS

M. VASTUS INTERNUS

M. TIBIALIS ANTICUS

M. PERONEUS LONGUS

M. EXTENSOR LONGUS DIGITORUM

M. PERONEUS BREVIS

M. EXTENSOR PROPRIUS POLLICIS

M. ABDUCTOR MINIMI DIGITI

M. EXTENSOR BREVIS DIGITORUM

MM. INTEROSSEI

M = Muscle
N = Nerves

M. GLUTEUS MAXIMUS

M. GLUTEUS MEDIUS

M. TENSOR VAGINAE FEMORIS

N. GREAT SCIATIC

MM. SEMITENDINOSUS AND SEMIMEMBRANOSUS

M. BICEPS

N. INTERNAL POPLITEAL (TIBIAL)

N. EXTERNAL POPLITEAL (PERONEAL)

M. GASTROCNEMIUS

M. SOLEUS

M. FLEXOR LONGUS DIGITORUM

M. FLEXOR LONGUS HALLUCIS

N. INTERNAL POPLITEAL (TIBIAL)

Labeling Key

■ Increased sensation with no associated muscle contraction

● Associated muscle contraction

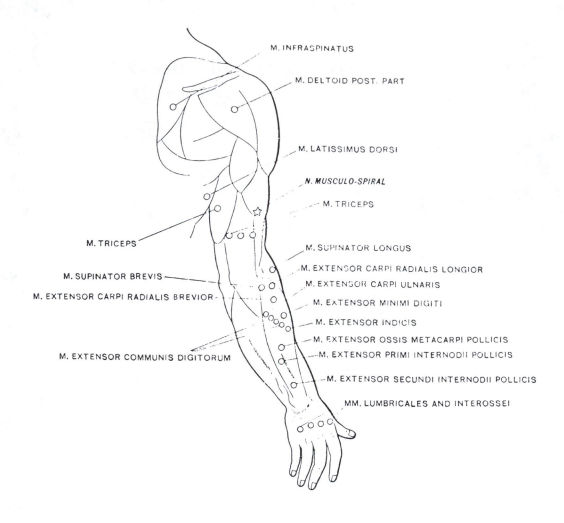

M. INFRASPINATUS

M. DELTOID POST. PART

M. LATISSIMUS DORSI

N. MUSCULO-SPIRAL

M. TRICEPS

M. TRICEPS

M. SUPINATOR LONGUS

M. EXTENSOR CARPI RADIALIS LONGIOR

M. SUPINATOR BREVIS

M. EXTENSOR CARPI ULNARIS

M. EXTENSOR CARPI RADIALIS BREVIOR

M. EXTENSOR MINIMI DIGITI

M. EXTENSOR INDICIS

M. EXTENSOR OSSIS METACARPI POLLICIS

M. EXTENSOR PRIMI INTERNODII POLLICIS

M. EXTENSOR COMMUNIS DIGITORUM

M. EXTENSOR SECUNDI INTERNODII POLLICIS

MM. LUMBRICALES AND INTEROSSEI

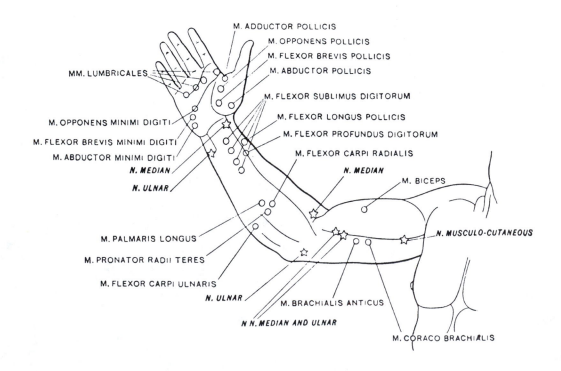

M. ADDUCTOR POLLICIS

M. OPPONENS POLLICIS

M. FLEXOR BREVIS POLLICIS

M. ABDUCTOR POLLICIS

MM. LUMBRICALES

M. FLEXOR SUBLIMUS DIGITORUM

M. OPPONENS MINIMI DIGITI

M. FLEXOR LONGUS POLLICIS

M. FLEXOR BREVIS MINIMI DIGITI

M. FLEXOR PROFUNDUS DIGITORUM

M. ABDUCTOR MINIMI DIGITI

M. FLEXOR CARPI RADIALIS

N. MEDIAN

N. MEDIAN

N. ULNAR

M. BICEPS

N. MUSCULO-CUTANEOUS

M. PALMARIS LONGUS

M. PRONATOR RADII TERES

M. FLEXOR CARPI ULNARIS

N. ULNAR

M. BRACHIALIS ANTICUS

N N. MEDIAN AND ULNAR

M. CORACO BRACHIALIS

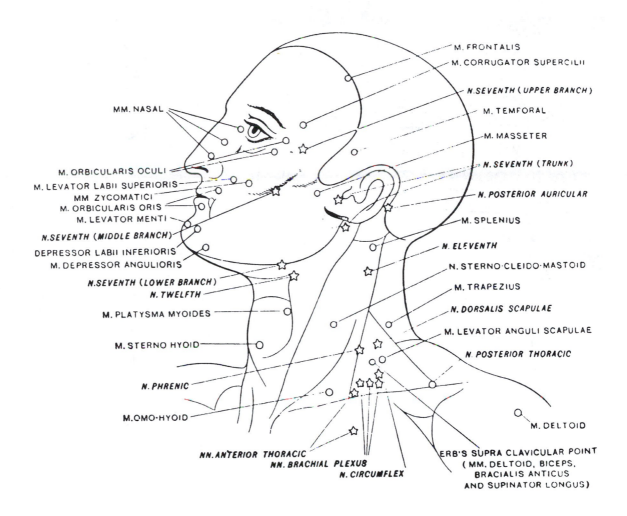

MM. NASAL

M. ORBICULARIS OCULI
M. LEVATOR LABII SUPERIORIS
MM ZYCOMATICI
M. ORBICULARIS ORIS
M. LEVATOR MENTI
N. SEVENTH (MIDDLE BRANCH)
DEPRESSOR LABII INFERIORIS
M. DEPRESSOR ANGULIORIS

N. SEVENTH (LOWER BRANCH)
N. TWELFTH

M. PLATYSMA MYOIDES

M. STERNO HYOID

N. PHRENIC

M. OMO-HYOID

NN. ANTERIOR THORACIC
NN. BRACHIAL PLEXUS
N. CIRCUMFLEX

M. FRONTALIS
M. CORRUGATOR SUPERCILII
N. SEVENTH (UPPER BRANCH)
M. TEMPORAL
M. MASSETER
N. SEVENTH (TRUNK)
N. POSTERIOR AURICULAR
M. SPLENIUS
N. ELEVENTH
N. STERNO-CLEIDO-MASTOID
M. TRAPEZIUS
N. DORSALIS SCAPULAE
M. LEVATOR ANGULI SCAPULAE
N. POSTERIOR THORACIC

M. DELTOID
ERB'S SUPRA CLAVICULAR POINT
(MM. DELTOID, BICEPS,
BRACIALIS ANTICUS
AND SUPINATOR LONGUS)

ACUPUNCTURE POINTS

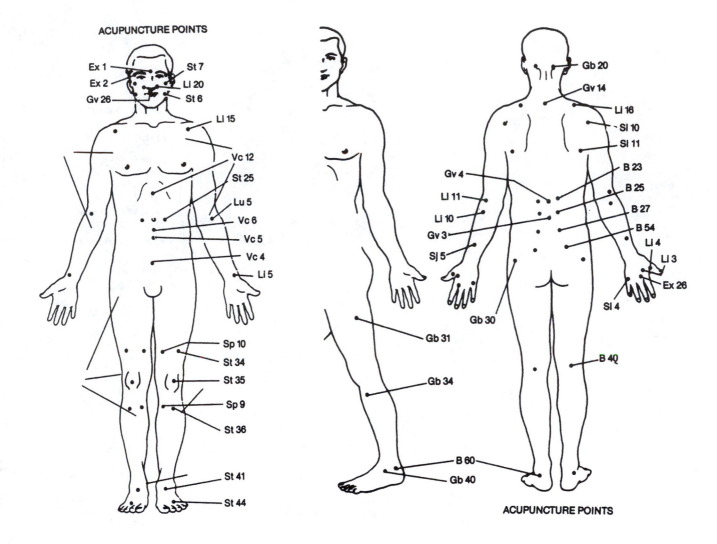

ACUPUNCTURE POINTS

▣ Activity Questions

1. Review your results from Activity 4–7. Were you able to elicit contractions from approximately the same locations on the body? To what do you attribute any difference?

2. What factor limited the maximal output intensity of the electrical stimulation device used in this activity?

Influence of Varying Electrical Stimulation Parameters

■ Objective

To become familiar with the various parameters available on electrical stimulators and how changing those parameters influences perception of the current.

■ Materials

- Various electrical stimulators (may include units with multiple-current types)
- Instruction manuals (including manufacturer specifications) for each stimulator

■ Procedures

1. Review the instruction manuals to determine the specifications for the unit (e.g., current types available, wave forms), and complete the chart appropriately.
2. Using the subject's forearm or thigh, configure the electrodes in a formation appropriate to the type of current being assessed.
3. Select an available parameter from the list below.

Possible Parameters	Sequence of Activity
Frequency:	High to low
Polarity:	Positive or negative
Pulse duration:	Long to short
Interpulse interval:	Short to long
Wave form:	Any sequence
Ramp time:	Zero to short to long
Current modulation:	Continuous frequency modulation amplitude modulation, multiple modulations
Sweep time:	Short to long

4. Increase the intensity until the subject feels a comfortably strong sensation, and note the intensity.
5. Reduce the intensity to zero, and vary the parameter in the direction indicated. Increase the intensity to the initial level.
6. Record the subject's comments about the different sensations in the space provided.
7. Repeat Steps 3 through 6 using a different parameter.

Note: If you are using a parameter not listed above, ask your instructor what sequence to use.

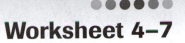
Influence of Varying Electrical Stimulation Parameters

Name: _____   Date: _____

Subject(s): _____

Name/Manufacturer of Stimulator: _____

Available Current Types:		
☐ Monophasic	☐ Biphasic	☐ Microcurrent
☐ Alternating	☐ Direct Current	☐ Interferential Current
Type of Current Used:		
Parameter Varied	Specifics: Tested	Comments (Perceptual change as parameter is varied)

Available Current Types:		
Monophasic	Biphasic	Microcurrent
Alternating Current	Direct Current	Interferential Current
Type of Current Used:		
Parameter Varied	Specifics Tested	Comments (Perceptual change as parameter is varied)

■ Activity Questions

1. Varying what single parameter most greatly influenced your perception of the current?

2. What combination of current parameters created the most comfortable current? The least comfortable?

3. For what purpose would a current ramp be used?

4. What is the benefit derived from modulating the current? Under what conditions is this parameter best used?

Medical Galvanism

Objective

To understand the difference in the migration of hydrogen and oxygen molecules between electrical modalities that use monophasic, biphasic, and direct currents.

Materials Needed

- Monophasic current stimulator (e.g., HVPS)
- Three beakers
- Biphasic stimulator (e.g., TENS)
- Distilled water
- Galvanic stimulator (iontophoresor)

Description of Galvanism

Through an electromotive force, ions may be attracted to or repelled from electrical poles. Similar to magnetic poles, negatively charged ions are attracted to the positive pole, whereas positively charged ions are repelled from it, and vice versa for the negative pole (Fig. 4–6). Several treatment approaches, such as controlling the formation of edema, are based on this principle, and the effectiveness is largely based on the type of current being used.

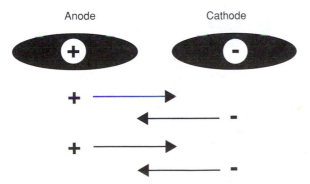

Anode   Cathode

Figure 4–6. Electromotive force, movement of ions.

Procedures

1. Using distilled (degassed) water, fill three beakers.
2. In the three beakers, secure the bare electrode leads (from each of the three stimulators) approximately 2 to 3 inches apart from each other. Ensure that the leads are not touching the sides of the beaker or each other.
3. For those units delivering pulsed currents, set the output parameters to the highest possible number of pulses per second and the longest pulse duration. This parameter is not applicable to direct current (DC) generators. Where applicable, ensure that the output is constant (not modulated) and that the unit is operating at a 100% duty cycle.
4. Increase the intensity to the maximal possible output.
5. Allow the current to run for 10 minutes. Do not disturb the units, beakers, or wires during the duration of this demonstration.
6. At the end of the 10-minute period, note the number and size of the bubbles that are clinging to each electrode. The larger hydrogen should be attracted to the cathode (negative pole) and oxygen bubbles to the anode (positive pole).

Notes

- Distilled water is available commercially, or tap water can be distilled by letting it sit uncovered for 24 hours.
- Prolonged use of stimulators using these parameters may result in damage to the equipment.
- Your observations should have demonstrated that the largest number and largest-sized bubbles were formed on the leads arising from the DC generator. The size and number of bubbles on the leads from the monophasic current should be significantly less than those found on the DC leads. No bubble formation should have been found on the leads emanating from the biphasic generator.

Medical Galvanism

Name: _____   Date: _____

Subject(s): _____

Electrode	Number of bubbles	Size of bubbles
Anode		
Cathode		

Activity Question

1. Iontophoresis involves the use of a galvanic current to introduce medications into the subcutaneous tissues. Based on your findings in this exercise, what would be the relationship between the ionic charge of the medications used during iontophoresis? What role would current polarity have? What would be the result if an electrically neutral medication were used?

Neuromuscular Strength Augmentation

Objectives

- To demonstrate the use of several forms of electrical stimulation to elicit a muscle contraction of the quadriceps muscle group.
- To appreciate the comfort levels and effectiveness of each form of electrical stimulation and how changing parameters and electrode configurations can influence the comfort level and effectiveness.

Materials Needed

- High-volt pulsed stimulator
- Neuromuscular electrical stimulator
- TENS unit
- Russian stimulator
- Electromagnetic or hydraulic isokinetic dynamometer or hand-held dynamometer

Measuring Electrically Induced Muscle Contractions

An electrical current can be used to evoke a muscle contraction. Several factors influence the quality of these contractions, including the type of current, pulse duration, pulse frequency, output intensity, and electrode placement. The intensity of these contractions may be measured quantitatively using commercially available isokinetic units by comparing the force produced by an electrically induced involuntary isometric contraction (IIC) to that obtained by a maximal voluntary isometric contraction (MVIC).

After locking the limb in the position to be tested, the subject performs a maximal isometric contraction of the quadriceps muscle, and the value is recorded. An electrical stimulation unit may then be configured to the extensor musculature, and the force of the contraction is again measured (Fig. 4–7). Note that when the leg is hanging on the dynamometer, the output will read in negative numbers (e.g., -14 ft-lb). This represents the force of gravity placing a force opposite that of the movement. Once the contraction, volun-

tary or involuntary, exceeds the force of gravity, these numbers will read as positive values.

The percentage of the MVIC obtained is determined by the formula: (IIC/MVIC) × 100.

Procedures

1. Use of an isokinetic unit is recommended for this activity. If not available, a hand-held dynamometer may be substituted.
2. Set up the isokinetic dynamometer for isometric knee extension testing at approximately 70° of flexion according to the manufacturer's instructions.
3. Using the protocol specific to the dynamometer used, determine the person's MVIC force.
4. Instructions for use of a hand-held dynamometer during testing are provided with each electrical stimulation unit. For specific directions on the use of a hand-held dynamometer, refer to the manufacturer's manual.

High-Volt Pulsed Stimulator

1. Establish the baseline strength of the subject by asking for a maximal voluntary isometric muscle contraction against the dynamometer placed over the anterior ankle of the subject.

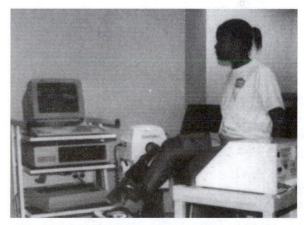

Figure 4–7. Set-up for testing force of contraction.

2. As high-volt pulsed stimulation uses a direct current, first decide what type of polarity will be used and what type of electrode configuration will be used. Begin with negative polarity and a monopolar electrode configuration. The smaller active electrode should be designated the negative pole. Place the dispersive electrode on the hamstrings or gastrocnemius of the same leg.

3. Place the active electrode over the motor point of the quadriceps muscle group after cleaning the area appropriately to reduce resistance.

4. Pulse frequency should be set at 10, 20, 40, 60, and 100 pps. Note the comfort level and effectiveness of contraction with the different frequencies.

5. Set the on and off time or duty cycle. For strengthening purposes, an on time of 10–15 seconds with an off time of 50 seconds to 2 minutes is warranted. Also attempt an on:off time of 5:5. Note the differences in fatigue after 5–10 minutes of treatment.

6. If pulse duration is variable within the machine, adjust it to 200–600 μsec.

7. Increase the intensity gradually according to the subject's responses.

8. Measure the torque produced by the electrically induced muscle contraction by using the hand-held dynamometer as before.

9. Ask the subject to rate the pain or comfort level on a VAS or 0–10 scale.

10. Adjust the parameters in Steps 2–6, and note comfort level changes and torque changes.

TENS Unit

1. As before, determine the baseline torque of the subject through the hand-held dynamometer and a maximal voluntary isometric contraction.

2. As most TENS units are alternating current (AC), the typical electrode configuration will be bipolar. Place the electrodes over the motor points of the quadriceps muscle group. You may alter the placement later to determine the most effective and comfortable placement.

3. Set the pulse frequency to 10, 20, 40, 60, and 100 pps. Note the comfort level and effectiveness of contraction with each frequency.

4. Set the on and off time or duty cycle. As with HVPS, the on and off time for strengthening is most effective at 10–15 seconds on and 1–2 minutes off. Adjust the on:off times later to determine the effect on fatigue and comfort.

5. Adjust pulse duration to the motor levels of 200–600 μsec. Also note the quality of the muscle contraction with pulse durations below 200 μsec.

6. Increase the intensity gradually according to the subject's responses.

7. Measure the torque produced by the electrically induced muscle contraction by using the hand-held dynamometer at the anterior ankle.

Russian Stimulator

1. Establish the baseline as before with an MVIC and the hand-held dynamometer.

2. Russian stimulators typically deliver medium-frequency (2000–10,000 Hz) wave carriers of polyphasic AC. Pulse duration and pulse frequency are usually adjustable. With AC, bipolar electrode configurations are typically used. Place the electrodes over the motor points of the quadriceps muscle group. Placement can be altered later to determine the most comfortable and most effective for muscle contractions.

3. Set the pulse frequencies at 10, 20, 40, 60, and 100 pps. Note the comfort level and effectiveness of contraction with the different frequencies.

4. Set the on and off time or duty cycle. On time of 10–15 seconds with off time of 1–2 minutes is warranted for strengthening purposes.

5. If pulse duration is adjustable within the machine, adjust it from 50–600 μsec, and note the quality of the muscle contraction and comfort level with each new setting.

6. Increase the intensity gradually according to the subject's responses.

7. Measure the torque produced by the electrically induced muscle contraction via the hand-held dynamometer.

8. Also note the comfort level with the VAS or 0–10 scale.

9. Adjust the parameters above, and note changes in muscle contractions and comfort levels.

Notes

- Allow sufficient time for muscle recovery between bouts.
- This activity may be modified by altering the output parameters and electrode placement as well as changing the position of the lower extremity.
- It is common for the subject to experience muscle soreness following this activity.

Neuromuscular Strength Augmentation

Name: _____ Date: _____

Subject(s): _____

Maximal Voluntary Isometric Contraction		
Subject	Joint Angle	Peak Torque

Subject	Electrical Stimulator	Electrode Configuration	Pulse Duration	Pulses Per Second	Duty Cycle	Max. Output Intensity	Pain (0–10)	Joint Angle	Peak Torque	%MVIC

Activity Questions

1. Based on the activity, would you expect a stronger contraction using a monopolar or bipolar pad arrangement?

2. Considering your results, which electrical stimulator would you use to obtain an optimal muscle contraction? Why?

3. Following a period of rest or using the opposite leg, determine the IIC using various duty cycles by altering the rest duration. What can be deduced from this activity regarding the implication of fatigue in electrically assisted muscle contractions?

4. You are attempting to strengthen the vastus medialis oblique with a bipolar set-up over the anterior thigh but are unable to elicit a muscle contraction before the subject complains of discomfort. What can you do to make the patient more comfortable and still elicit a muscle contraction?

Effect of Cold Application in Reducing the Perception of Electrically Induced Pain

◼ Objective

To determine if cold application before or during electrical stimulation reduces the individual's perception of pain.

◼ Materials Needed

- High-volt pulsed stimulator
- Interferential electrical stimulator
- TENS unit
- Russian stimulator

◼ Procedures

1. Using a monopolar electrode configuration, attach the "dispersive" electrode on the subject's lower back or thigh and the "active" electrode to the anterior portion of the subject's forearm (this configuration is recommended for high-volt pulsed units). If other stimulators are used, arrange the electrodes in a bipolar configuration, placing one electrode on the distal portion of the subject's anterior forearm and the other on the proximal portion of the anterior forearm.
2. Set the stimulation parameters to the following values. (It is recommended that the final parameters from Activity 4–2, Selective Stimulation of Nerves, also be used so that the results of these two exercises can be compared.)

Parameters	Settings
Pulse duration:	60 μsec
Pulse frequency:	30 pps
Pad alternating rate:	Continuous
Modulation parameters:	Off (constant output)
Duty cycle:	100%

Note: Not all parameters will be applicable to each unit.

3. Slowly increase the intensity until pain is experienced. Do not let the subject watch the output meter. Note and record the output intensity.
4. Reduce the intensity, remove the electrodes from the subject's forearm, and turn the generator off.
5. Apply a cold modality to the forearm until numbness is reported.
6. Reattach the electrodes, and reapply the cold modality to the forearm.
7. Slowly increase the intensity until the subject reports pain. Note and record the output intensity.
8. Repeat this activity using multiple subjects, or obtain the values obtained by other groups.
9. Statistical analysis, such as the t-Test, may be used to determine if there is a significant difference between pain perception with and without concurrent cold application.

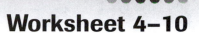

Effect of Cold Application in Reducing the Perception of Electrically Induced Pain

Name: _____   Date: _____

Subject(s): _____

Type of Stimulator Used: _____

Maximum Output Intensity			
Subject	No Cold Application	With Cold Application	Difference

▮ Activity Questions

1. Did the intensity at which pain was reported increase or decrease after the cold application?

2. Based on the results of this exercise, how would you explain the findings of the two research studies cited (Miller and Webers, 1990; Durst et al, 1991) in the introduction of Unit 4?

Pain Control Using Electrical Stimulation

Objective

To determine comfort of different electrical stimulation units and the different parameters used to control pain.

Materials Needed

- High-volt pulsed stimulator
- Interferential electrical stimulator
- TENS unit

Procedures

1. Clean the area appropriately to reduce resistance.
2. Set the parameters for pain control using the charts below.
3. Increase the intensity gradually according to the subject's responses.
4. Ask the subject to rate their pain or comfort level on a VAS or 0–10 scale.
5. Use several different pain control settings and record the treatment parameters and subject comfort score on the chart provided.

High-Volt Pulsed Stimulator			
Parameters	**Gate control mechanism**	**Opiate release mechanism**	**Brief-intense protocol**
Output intensity	Sensory level	Motor level	Noxious
Pulse frequency	60–100 pps	2–4 pps	>120 pps
Phase duration	<100 μsec	150–250 μsec	>300 μsec
Mode	Continuous	Continuous	Probe (15–60 sec per site)
Electrode arrangement	Monopolar or bipolar	Monopolar or bipolar	Monopolar (probe)
Polarity	Acute: positive; Chronic: negative	Acute: positive; Chronic: negative	Acute: positive; Chronic: negative
Electrode placement	Directly over the painful site	Directly over the painful site, distal to the spinal nerve root origin, trigger points, or acupuncture points	Gridding technique

Note: Not all parameters will be applicable to each unit.

TENS			
Parameters	**High-frequency TENS**	**Low-frequency TENS**	**Brief-intense TENS**
Output intensity	Sensory level	Motor level	Noxious
Pulse frequency	60–100 pps	2–4 pps	Variable
Phase duration	60–100 μsec	150–250 μsec	300–1000 μsec
Mode	Modulated	Modulated	Modulated
Electrode arrangement	Direct or continuous	Direct or continuous	Direct or continuous

Note: Not all parameters will be applicable to each unit.

Interferential Stimulation		
Parameters	**Gate control**	**Opiate release**
Carrier frequency	Based on patient comfort	Based on patient comfort
Burst frequency	80–150 Hz	1–10 Hz
Sweep	Fast	Slow
Electrode arrangement	Quadripolar	Quadripolar
Electrode placement	Around the periphery of the target area	Around the periphery of the target area
Output intensity	Strong sensory level	Moderate to strong sensory level

Note: Not all parameters will be applicable to each unit.

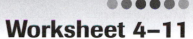

Pain Control Using Electrical Stimulation

Name: _____ Date: _____

Subject(s): _____

Comfort Scale

Very
Comfortable   Extremely
                                                              Uncomfortable

0   1   2   3   4   5   6   7   8   9   10

Using the comfort scale provided, complete the following table by writing the comfort score in the space provided.

Subject	Stimulator/Treatment parameters	Comfort score (0–10)

Activity Questions

1. Which unit and set-up appeared to be the most comfortable? Which was the most uncomfortable?

2. If you were planning to treat an elderly patient with chronic pain and the patient seemed apprehensive to the use of electrical stimulation, what unit and treatment protocol might be the most appropriate? What could you do to prepare the patient for the treatment and calm the concerns about electrical stimulation?

Edema Reduction Using Electrical Stimulation

Objective

To demonstrate knowledge of the characteristics associated with different electrical stimulation units and the different parameters used to control edema.

Materials Needed

- High-volt pulsed stimulator
- Neuromuscular electrical stimulator

Procedures

1. Clean the area appropriately to reduce resistance.
2. Set the parameters for edema reduction using the chart below.
3. Properly support and elevate the injured area.
4. Apply a compression wrap, if indicated, to the injured region.
5. Increase the intensity gradually according to the subject's responses.
6. Use several different edema reduction settings.

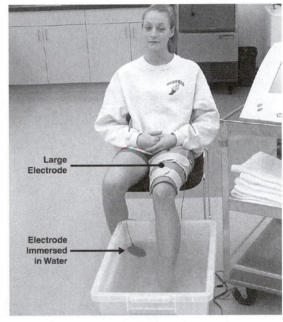

Large Electrode

Electrode Immersed in Water

Figure 4–8. Treatment set up for sensory-level control of edema formation using the immersion method.

Parameters	High-volt pulsed stimulator: Sensory-level	High-volt pulsed stimulator: Motor-level	Neuromuscular electrical stimulator: Motor-level
Output intensity	Sensory level	Motor level	Motor level
Pulse frequency	120 pps	2–4 pps	1–10 pps
Pulse duration	Maximum allowed by generator		
Mode	Continuous	Alternating	Continuous (On: off—100% duty cycle)
Electrode arrangement	Immersion method (Fig. 4–8) or active electrodes around injured tissues	Monopolar or bipolar	Bipolar
Polarity	Negative	Positive or negative	
Electrode placement	Electrodes placed over injured tissue	Bipolar: proximal and distal ends of the muscle just proximal to the edema region. Monopolar: active electrodes along path of venous return.	Proximal and distal ends of the muscle just proximal to the edema region.
Comments	Begin this procedure as quickly as possible following the trauma. This procedure should not be used if significant swelling is already present.	Review status of the injury. Make sure the treatment will not induce excessive joint movement that might be contraindicated.	Review status of the injury. Make sure the treatment will not induce excessive joint movement that might be contraindicated.

Note: Not all parameters will be applicable to each unit.

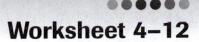

Edema Reduction Using Electrical Stimulation

Name: _____   Date: _____

Subject(s): _____

■ Activity Questions

1. Interferential electrical stimulation can be used to treat edema formation. What would be the parameters that would be set when using interferential for the control of edema?

2. Could you use a neuromuscular electrical stimulation unit set with a higher frequency and 50% duty cycle to treat a patient for edema reduction? Support your answer.

3. The use of ice is recommended for the treatment of swelling. Is it appropriate to use ice when treating your patient with a high-volt pulsed stimulator for motor-level control of edema? Why or why not?

On completion of the activities for Unit 4, review the following case studies to enhance practical application of electrical modalities.

1. Following a 6-week immobilization of an ankle fracture, a cross-country runner is in need of peroneal strengthening. Which type of electrical stimulation would you use? Describe the set-up parameters for the treatment.

2. A laborer is being treated for lateral epicondylitis and displays weakened grip strength. You decide to use HVPS. Describe the parameters you would use. Also decide what type of electrode configuration you would use.

3. Explain the differences in duty cycle or on-time and off-time you would use if you were concentrating on increasing muscular endurance for the external rotators of a college pitcher or if you were concentrating on increasing muscular strength of the gastrocnemius of a college wrestler.

4. Your patient is a 56-year-old man with severe pain and decreased range of motion of his left shoulder. The pain is diffuse over a large portion of his shoulder. His pain appears to be secondary to a deltoid strain suffered 2 weeks ago while he was doing yard work. Describe the treatment options you have for treating this patient's chief complaint of pain.

5. Your patient is a 35-year-old tennis player with elbow tendonitis. He has been doing conservative treatment for 3 weeks, with little improvement in the tendonitis. He wants to play in a community tournament in 2 weeks. Your facility has the equipment to provide iontophoresis. Is this a good choice for treating this condition? If you choose to use iontophoresis, what is the set-up for the treatment? Be sure to include all necessary parameters.

Deep Heat Modalities

Background and Discussion

Deep heat treatments are administered through the use of ultrasound or shortwave diathermy. Deep heat application is indicated under these conditions: (1) to control the inflammatory reaction in its subacute or chronic stage, (2) to encourage tissue healing, (3) to reduce edema and ecchymosis, (4) to improve range of motion before physical activity or rehabilitation, or (5) to promote drainage from an infected site. Deep heating agents provide a longer-lasting effect than superficial heating agents.

Therapeutic ultrasound uses high-frequency sound waves applied to the body to induce tissue temperature increases. Ultrasound produces thermal and nonthermal physiological changes within deep tissues. Because ultrasonic energy cannot be transmitted through the air, a coupling medium must be used to transmit the sound waves to the tissues. All commercially available approved coupling gels meet this criterion. However, many times clinicians will substitute other forms of media, especially during phonophoresis treatments. Many of the different media with which hydrocortisone is mixed are totally incapable of transmitting ultrasonic energy. Likewise, many other phonophoresis media, such as Theragesic® or Aspercreme, have little or no ability to transmit ultrasound. Generally speaking, thick, white creams (such as hand/skin creams) are poor conductors, whereas gel-mixed agents serve as good conductors.[17] The gel pad, used with and without standard coupling gel, is also an efficient coupling agent.[18]

Shortwave diathermy is a high-frequency electromagnetic modality that can cause deep-tissue temperature increases. Like ultrasound, shortwave diathermy can evoke thermal and nonthermal tissue changes. The volume of tissue that can be heated during shortwave diathermy treatments is greater than the volume treated during ultrasound treatments. There are two types of shortwave diathermy: induction field generators and capacitive generators. The tissues that can be treated differ between the two generators. Generally, induction generators increase tissue temperature within the muscle layer, whereas capacitive generators heat the tissue directly under each plate. Thus, the treatment given depends on the generator type and set-up.

Contraindications

- Acute injuries
- Ischemic areas
- Impaired circulation
- Poor thermal regulation
- Anesthetic areas
- Already existing fever
- Malignancies
- Cardiac insufficiency
- Extremely old adults and children younger than 4 years
- Pregnancy
- Eyes

Additional contraindications specific to ultrasound:
- Pacemaker
- Central nervous system tissue
- Joint cement
- Implants with plastic components
- Immature epiphyseal plates (precaution)
- Fractures (precaution)

Additional contraindications specific to diathermy:
- Neural stimulators
- Metal implants (Note that the presence of metal in the body is device-dependent. In some cases, treatment can be provided.)
- Immature epiphyseal plates
- Obesity (precaution)
- Copper-type IUD
- Body piercings
- Electronic or magnetic equipment in the treatment area

Ultrasound Parameters Worksheet

■ Objective

To display a mastery of the concepts associated with thera-peutic ultrasound.

■ Definition of Terms

Beam Nonuniformity Ratio (BNR): The ratio between the spatial peak intensity to the average output as reported on unit's meter.

Duty Cycle: The ratio between the ultrasound's pulse length and pulse interval when ultrasound is being delivered in the pulsed mode.

Effective Radiating Area (ERA): The area of the ultra-sound head that produces mechanical waves, normally measured in square centimeters (cm^2).

Near Field: The portion of the ultrasound beam that is used for therapeutic purposes.

Spatial Average Intensity (SAI): The amount of ultrasound energy passing through the ultrasound head, expressed in watts per square centimeter (W/cm^2)

Spatial Peak Intensity (SPI): The maximum output (power) produced within an ultrasound beam.

Temporal Average Intensity (TAI): The power of ultrasonic output over a period of time. This measure is only mean-ingful with pulsed ultrasound.

Ultrasound: Mechanical sound waves occurring at fre-quency above the range of human hearing ($>20,000$ Hz). Therapeutic ultrasound ranges between 1 and 3 MHz.

■ Exercises

(Show your work for all calculations.)

1. Using an ultrasound unit having a 4:1 BNR, the me-tered output indicates that an average of 4 watts of power is being delivered to the tissues. What is the peak intensity being delivered to the tissues in this treatment?

2. The spatial average intensity of an ultrasound treatment depends on the ERA of the sound head. Calculate the output, in W/cm^2, for an ultrasound beam at an inten-sity of 5 watts for the following sound heads, each having a different ERA:

ERA	W/cm^2
10 cm^2	
8 cm^2	
5 cm^2	
3 cm^2	
1 cm^2	

3. Using the parameters cited below, calculate the percent duty cycle and the temporal average intensity, assum-ing that the metered output displays 4 W/cm^2:

10	10
20	40
10	50
25	60

4. The treatment duration and intensity of ultrasound treatment are frequently insufficient to achieve the desired therapeutic effects. Using the tables below and assuming a treatment area of two to three times the ERA, calculate the duration of the treatment for the desired effect:

Classification of US Heating	
Effect	Net Temperature Increase
Nonthermal	None
Mild thermal	1° C
Moderate thermal	2° C
Vigorous	4° C

US Heating Rate per Minute		
Intensity (W/cm^2)	1MHz	3 MHz
0.5	0.4° C	0.3° C
1.0	0.2° C	0.6° C
1.5	0.3° C	0.9° C
2.0	0.4° C	1.4° C

Tables adapted from Draper, DO: Ten mistakes commonly made with ultrasound use: Current research sheds light on myths. *Athletic Training: Sports Health Care Perspectives,* 2:98–99, 1996.

A. **Patellar tendinitis (vigorous heating desired)**

Ultrasound frequency:

Treatment duration at intensity of 0.5 W/cm^2:

Treatment duration at intensity of 1.0 W/cm^2:

Treatment duration at intensity of 2.0 W/cm^2:

B. **Chronic quadriceps contusion (mild heating desired)**

Ultrasound frequency:

Treatment duration at intensity of 1.0 W/cm^2:

Treatment duration at intensity of 2.0 W/cm^2:

Coupling Ability of Various Ultrasound Media

Objective

To determine the relative ability of various media to transmit ultrasonic energy.

Materials Needed

- Ultrasound unit(s) (with different size sound heads, if available)
- Athletic tape or similar
- Various ultrasound transmission media (e.g., commercial transmission gels, hydrocortisone mixtures, topical counterirritants, petroleum jelly)
- Bucket
- Plastic bag
- Latex glove

Procedures

1. Configure the ultrasound unit to continuous output and, if adjustable, the output meter to total watts (W).
2. Using athletic tape (or something similar), form a well around the ultrasound head (Fig. 5–1).
3. Fill the well with water.
4. Turn the unit on, and slowly increase the intensity until a steady movement (bubbling or agitation) of the water is seen.
5. Record the output intensity in W, and reset the unit.
6. For ease of application, remove the tape, and completely cover the ultrasound head with an even layer of coupling gel. Re-form the well with tape, and fill with water. Repeat Steps 4 and 5.
7. Repeat the process using different coupling media.
8. Repeat this exercise using a sound head of a different size.

Water Immersion

1. Fill a bucket/ceramic tub with water (preferably distilled water).
2. Place the ultrasound head in the tub.
3. Have the subject place a foot/hand into the tub.
4. Be sure to hold the sound head approximately 1 inch from the body part. Wipe off any air bubbles present on the sound head.
5. The dosage should be increased approximately 0.5 W/cm^2.

Bladder Method

1. Fill a balloon, plastic bag, or glove (bladder) with water, and coat with ultrasound gel. Be sure to remove any air bubbles. A gel pad may be used for this procedure.
2. Apply ultrasound gel to the body part.
3. Place the bladder or gel pad over the body part to be treated.
4. Apply the ultrasound head to the bladder or gel pad, and move over the bladder.

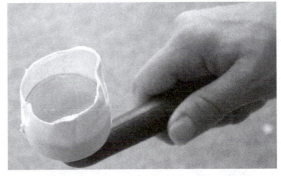

Figure 5–1.   Ultrasound head with athletic tape to form well.

■ Notes

- If available, a commercial ultrasound output meter (such as those used for calibrating the instrument) may be used.
- Practice caution if using older ultrasound generators that do not have an automatic shut-off feature built in.

Continually running the machine when the energy is not being transmitted (such as holding the transducer in the air and turning up the intensity) may seriously damage the crystal.

Coupling Ability of Various Ultrasound Media

Name: _____   Date: _____

Subject(s): _____

Coupling Medium	ERA	Wattage Needed to Produce Bubbles

■ Activity Questions

1. Which medium served as the best conductor of ultrasonic energy? Why?

2. Which medium appeared to be the least effective conductor of ultrasonic energy? Why?

3. Many of the media customarily used as bases for phonophoresis are not good conductors of ultrasonic energy, yet many individuals still report benefits from the treatment. Why might this occur?

4. How did your results change when a different size sound head was used? (If a different size sound head was not available, hypothesize the results.)

Ultrasound–Thermal and Nonthermal Treatments

Objective

To determine differences in patient sensation between thermal (changes within the tissues as a direct result of ultrasound's elevation of the tissue temperature) and nonthermal (changes within the tissues resulting from the mechanical effect of ultrasonic energy) ultrasound.

Materials Needed

- Ultrasound unit(s) (with 1 MHz capability)
- Ultrasound gel

Procedures

1. Establish that no contraindications to the use of ultrasound are present.
2. Configure the ultrasound unit to continuous output (100% duty cycle).
3. Choose a large muscle mass area to be treated. Clean the area to be treated. Apply ultrasound gel to the region. Be sure to identify a treatment area that is only 2 to 3 times the ERA of the unit you are using.
4. Turn the unit on, and slowly increase the intensity while moving the sound head. Increase the intensity to approximately 1.5 W/cm^2.
5. Move the sound head at a moderate pace, being sure to overlap your strokes.
6. At minutes 1 through 5, record the sensations described by your partner.
7. Stop treatment after 5 minutes.
8. Using the contralateral limb, repeat Step 3.
9. Configure the ultrasound unit to a 20% duty cycle.
10. Increase the intensity to 0.5 W/cm^2.
11. Repeat Steps 5 through 7.
12. On completing all procedures, remove any remaining ultrasound gel from the skin, and clean the sound head of the unit.

Ultrasound—Thermal and Nonthermal Treatments

Name: _____   Date: _____

Subject(s): _____

Treatment 1 (100% duty cycle; 1.5 W/cm^2)		
Time	**Skin sensations**	**Deep-tissue sensations**
Minute 1		
Minute 2		
Minute 3		
Minute 4		
Minute 5		

Treatment 2 (20% duty cycle; 0.5 W/cm^2)		
Time	**Skin sensations**	**Deep-tissue sensations**
Minute 1		
Minute 2		
Minute 3		
Minute 4		
Minute 5		

Activity Questions

1. Which provided the greatest warmth or heating feeling?

2. If a patient reports a feeling of discomfort (excessive heating) during treatment, should you always stop treatment? Or what measures can you take to correct this situation and continue the treatment?

3. Is the patient's information about the warming sensation felt to be an accurate reflection of the temperature increase within the muscle?

4. To ensure proper treatment in subsequent treatment sessions, what information should be recorded in the patient file?

Shortwave Diathermy

◼ Objective

To determine differences in patient sensation between thermal and nonthermal treatments with shortwave diathermy.

◼ Materials Needed

- Shortwave diathermy unit(s) (inductive drum and capacitive plate generators, if available)
- Towels

◼ Procedures

1. Establish that no contraindications to the use of shortwave diathermy are present.
2. Remove all jewelry and other metal items from your laboratory partner. The clinician should remove all personal jewelry. Be sure your laboratory partner will not come in contact with objects directly grounded (pipes, outlets, etc).
3. Choose a large muscle mass area to be treated. Clean and dry the area to be treated.
4. Cover the area to be treated with a dry terry-cloth towel.
5. Turn the unit on. Allow time for the unit to warm up, if necessary. Follow the manufacturer's directions for "tuning" the generator.
6. Set the drum or plates properly to ensure positioning is uniform between the unit and the tissue area being treated.
7. Set the timer to the desired time (5 minutes for this laboratory experiment).
8. Increase the intensity until your laboratory partner feels mild warmth. Set the unit to a low average intensity and an output of less than 38 W.
9. Check the area frequently for signs of excessive heating or burns.
10. Record information about the treatment on the table provided (nonthermal).
11. Repeat Steps 2 through 9 with a higher average intensity and an output of greater than 38 W.
12. Record information about the treatment on the table provided (thermal treatment).
13. On completing all procedures, clean the unit following the manufacturer's specifications.

Shortwave Diathermy—Thermal and Nonthermal Treatments

Name: _____   Date: _____

Subject(s): _____

Treatment 1 (low average intensity and an output of less than 38 W)		
Time	Skin sensations	Deep-tissue sensations
Minute 1		
Minute 2		
Minute 3		
Minute 4		
Minute 5		

Treatment 2 (higher average intensity and an output of greater than 38 W)		
Time	Skin sensations	Deep-tissue sensations
Minute 1		
Minute 2		
Minute 3		
Minute 4		
Minute 5		

▇ Activity Questions

1. Did you feel mild warmth during both treatments?

2. Compare the treatment sensations with those from the ultrasound laboratory activity (Activity 5–3). Which technique (ultrasound or shortwave diathermy) could treat a larger area? Did one of the treatments seem to have a faster response with respect to tissue temperature increase?

3. If a patient reports a feeling of discomfort (excessive heating) during treatment, should you always stop treatment? Or can you take measures to correct this situation and continue the treatment?

4. To ensure proper treatment in subsequent treatment sessions, what treatment parameters should be recorded in the patient file?

On completion of the activities for Unit 5, review the following case studies to enhance practical application of superficial heat modalities.

1. If you had a patient referred to you for treatment of chronic patellar tendonitis, which deep heating method(s) would you use? Why? What contraindications must you address for the modality you chose? Would you change your treatment plan if the tendonitis was considered acute or subacute?

2. You are preparing to treat a 21-year-old athlete diagnosed with Achilles tendonitis, and you wish to use ultrasound. What treatment method would you use? Which parameters would you use? Why?

3. A-28-year-old auto mechanic was referred to you for treatment. He is complaining of nagging back pain that has progressively worsened over the last month. He presents with a slight decrease in lumbar lordosis, generalized pain throughout the lumbar spine, no palpable tenderness, and slight active range of motion deficits. You perform an initial evaluation and determine no specific pathology or malalignment. Your initial treatment goals are decreasing the back pain and increasing range of motion. What are your best choices for modalities? Consider contraindications in your decisions. Would your choice of treatment change if your patient had previously had back surgery and has metal implants?

Mechanical Modalities

■ Background and Discussion

This unit will provide laboratory experiences on mechanical modalities. These modalities rely on mechanical forces to impact the injury response process.

Intermittent compression units apply pressure to the body to enhance venous and lymphatic flow. The primary purpose for the use of intermittent compression is to force fluids and solids from the injury site to reduce edema. Spreading the edema over a larger area increases the lymphatic system's ability to absorb and remove the exudates. The units function to provide either circumferential (equal pressure to all parts of extremity) or sequential (distal to proximal) compression. The compression is applied to an extremity by way of air or cold water flowing through a sleeve device that is fitted over the extremity.

Surface electromyography (EMG) cannot directly measure the force of a muscle contraction. However, surface EMG biofeedback can assess the electrical correlate to a muscle contraction and provide this information to the user in the form of visual and/or auditory feedback. EMG biofeedback units typically have three electrodes, with two used to gather information from the muscle and the third acting as a reference electrode, filtering unwanted information.

Biofeedback is ideally used early in the rehabilitation process to reestablish neurological pathways lost because of immobilization or nerve damage. Even though healthy muscle will be used in the activities in this Unit, the concept of monitoring electrical activity in the muscle is the same. If we were attempting to reeducate unhealthy or unused muscle, the procedures and principles would remain the same; only a lower threshold would be used. Thus, the biofeedback unit is being used as a learning tool to increase the subject's awareness and subsequently assist in the neural development of the pathways necessary to contract a muscle. Because the final goal of EMG biofeedback is unassisted voluntary contraction, the final phase of each treatment session should conclude with an exercise bout without the assistance of feedback.

Therapeutic massage is a mechanical modality that can elicit numerous responses (invigorate or relax), depending on the procedure used. While the beneficial effects of massage may be partially psychological, it has been demonstrated to be effective in reduction of edema, reducing muscle spasm, and decreasing pain.

Traction, or more accurately distraction, is used to separate the bony elements of the spine and to elongate the associated soft tissues in the spinal region. Until recently, traction was used primarily to treat fractures, dislocations, and deformities of the spine and the extremities. It is now used to manage specific disorders of the spine. Research has shown that traction can effectively increase the space between the vertebral bodies, the articulating facets, and the intervertebral foramen. Traction is effective in promoting relaxation of paraspinal musculature, reducing the bulging of a herniated disc, and reducing the pressure on nerve roots in the intervertebral foramen. Many types of traction can be utilized but are beyond the scope of this laboratory manual. We will concentrate on intermittent mechanical traction and manual traction of the cervical and lumbar spine. Intermittent mechanical traction uses a mechanical device that alternately applies and releases traction for short intervals (usually 15–60 seconds). Manual traction is applied by the athletic trainer, physical therapist, or family member. It can also be used as a diagnostic tool to determine if traction will be beneficial for the patient. Note that to reduce the risk of injury, the lowest amount of traction force needed to obtain therapeutic effects should be used. Increased forces result in increased risk of injury. Proper evaluation of the integrity of the cervical ligaments and vertebral arteries should be performed. Ensure tinnitus, nystagmus, nausea, visual changes, and dizziness do not occur before proceeding with traction.

Continuous passive motion devices (CPM) are available in three forms: free linkage, anatomic, and nonanatomic. Each type of CPM device has strengths and weaknesses with respect to individual characteristics. The main reasons for the use of a CPM unit is to maintain motion to stimulate healing through increased metabolic activity on articular cartilage, decrease edema, and improve nutrition throughout the joint via improved synovial fluid movement. Thus, the continuous, light stress applied to the joint is purported to decrease edema and enhance remodeling of collagen fibers.

Contraindications specific to intermittent compression

- Acute injuries with possibility of fracture
- Conditions in which pressure could result in increased tissue damage
- Poor thermal regulation
- Anesthetic areas
- Peripheral vascular disease
- Arteriosclerosis
- Edema secondary to congestive heart failure
- Ischemic vascular disease
- Gangrene
- Dermatitis
- Deep vein thrombosis (DVT)
- Thrombophlebitis

Contraindications specific to massage

- Acute injuries or inflammation
- Open wounds, skin conditions
- Fracture sites
- Impaired circulation
- Swelling caused by kidney or liver disease, cardiovascular insufficiency, or pleural effusion

Contraindications specific to traction

- Any local or systemic disease affecting the joints, ligaments, bones, and muscles such as tumors, infections, rheumatoid arthritis, and osteoporosis. The quality of these structures may not be strong enough to sustain the high forces utilized in traction.
- Unstable spine
- Diseases affecting the vertebra or spinal cord, including cancer and meningitis
- Vertebral fractures
- Extruded disc fragmentation
- Spinal cord compression
- Any condition in which vertebral flexion and/or extension is contraindicated
- Osteoporosis
- Conditions that worsen during and after traction treatments

Contraindications specific to continuous passive motion

- Unwanted joint motion
- Unstable fractures
- Areas of infection
- DVT (precaution)
- Spastic paralyses

Intermittent Compression

Objective

To demonstrate the proper set-up and use of an intermittent compression device.

Materials Needed

- Intermittent compression unit (Fig. 6–1)
- Blood pressure cuff and stethoscope
- Tape measure

Procedures

1. Review and ensure the patient does not have contraindications for the use of intermittent compression.

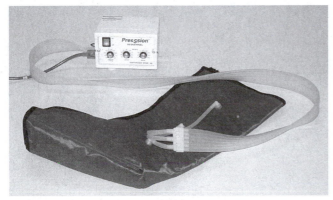

Figure 6–1. Intermittent compression unit.

2. Remove any tight clothing or jewelry from the extremity to be treated.
3. Measure the blood pressure of the patient to determine diastolic blood pressure.
4. Mark two areas on the extremity to measure the circumference of the extremity in the area to be treated. Measure the circumference, and record it on the chart provided.
5. Cover the area to be treated with Stockinette, making sure the area is free of wrinkles.
6. Apply the sleeve device to the extremity, and elevate the extremity.
7. Connect the hoses from the motorized compression unit to the sleeve. Ensure the hoses are connected properly.
8. Select the temperature to be used for the treatment.
9. Select the pressure for the treatment (upper extremity: 40–60 mm Hg; lower extremity: 60 to 100 mm Hg). In most cases the pressure should not exceed the diastolic pressure of the patient.
10. Set the on:off time using a 3:1 ratio.
11. Set the treatment time for 10 minutes (usual treatment duration is 20–30 minutes).
12. Monitor the patient for sensations related to the treatment. If appropriate, instruct the patient to perform gentle range-of-motion exercises during the treatment.
13. On completion of the treatment, switch the unit to drain mode to drain the fluid.
14. Remove the sleeve from the extremity.
15. Remeasure the extremity at the two locations identified in Step 4, and record the measurements on the chart.

Intermittent Compression

Name: _____ Date: _____

Subject(s): _____

Measurement location	Pretreatment measurement	Post-treatment measurement
Proximal mark		
Distal mark		

Sensations

During application (minute 5)

_____

End of application (minute 10)

_____

▮ Activity Questions

1. Following an intermittent compression treatment, would you recommend the use of a compression wrap? Why or why not?

2. Intermittent compression is contraindicated in cases in which the patient has DVT. However, it is indicated for the prevention of DVT. What special procedures might you implement when using intermittent compression for prevention of DVT?

Strength of Biofeedback-Augmented Muscle Contractions

Objective

To determine the effectiveness of visual and/or auditory biofeedback, or both, in increasing voluntary isometric contraction of the quadriceps muscle group.

Materials Needed

- Single-channel biofeedback unit
- Electromagnetic or hydraulic isokinetic device or hand-held grip dynamometer.

Procedures

1. See Activity 4–9, Neuromuscular Strength Augmentation, for a description of measuring the strength of muscle contractions.

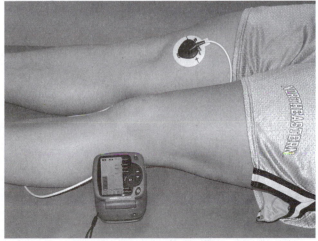

Figure 6–2.   Placement of electrode over the vastus medialis.

2. Set up the dynamometer for isometric knee extension testing at approximately 15° of flexion according to the manufacturer's instructions.
3. Using the protocol specific to the dynamometer being used, determine the subject's maximal voluntary isometric contraction (MVIC) force. Record this value on the chart provided.
4. Using the recommended coupling medium, attach the three biofeedback electrodes to the oblique fibers of the vastus medialis, making sure that the "active" electrodes are directly over the muscle belly. (Fig. 6–2) (The "reference" electrode is commonly black or red and is often placed to form a triangle with the two active electrodes.)
5. Find the threshold EMG level that the subject can achieve only through near-maximal isometric contraction.
6. Select one of three biofeedback parameters: (a) metered feedback only, (b) audio feedback only, or (c) both metered and audio feedback.
7. Measure the MVIC produced in conjunction with each of the three feedback methods described in Step 6.

Notes

- If a biofeedback unit is not available, perform this exercise in two bouts, one in which the subject cannot see the dynamometer's output display and one in which the subject can see the display.
- Muscle soreness may be experienced following the completion of this activity.
- If an isokinetic unit is not available, this activity can be performed using a hand-held grip dynamometer and fixing the biofeedback electrodes over the muscle bellies of the long finger flexors.

Strength of Biofeedback-Augmented Muscle Contractions

Name: _____   Date: _____

Subject(s): _____

Subject	No Feedback (%)	Visual Feedback (%)	Audible Feedback (%)	Both (%)

Activity Questions

1. Under which condition, if any, was the baseline MVIC exceeded?

2. Explain the similarities and differences between biofeedback and other feedback types (e.g., touching the muscle, yelling encouragement).

3. Would you raise or lower the threshold if you were targeting a smaller muscle, such as the abductor digiti minimi?

Educating Muscle Using Biofeedback

Objective

To understand the principles and effects of educating muscle through EMG biofeedback by eliciting a voluntary unilateral eyebrow raise.

Materials Needed

- EMG biofeedback
- Mirror

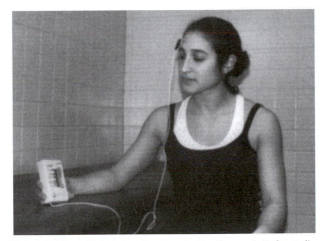

Figure 6–3.   Electrode placement over the occipitofrontalis.

Procedures

1. Place the electrodes over the occipitofrontalis muscle located above one of the eyebrows (Fig. 6–3).
2. Adjust the biofeedback threshold to the lowest sensitivity level that does not produce feedback of electrical activity at rest.
3. Position the mirror (or provide verbal feedback) so the subject will be aware of a unilateral rather than a bilateral raising of the eyebrow.
4. Continue to decrease the sensitivity of the biofeedback unit as the subject's muscle becomes educated to the contraction.
5. Once the subject learns how to accomplish this task, remove the electrodes, and have the subject attempt to raise an eyebrow without the assistance of biofeedback.

Note

- If the subject can already perform a unilateral eyebrow raise, attempt to elicit a contraction from another rarely used muscle such as the auricularis superior, which raises the ear superiorly and posteriorly.

Activity Questions

1. During the early stages of this exercise, it is not uncommon for both eyebrows to rise. To what neurophysiological principle do you attribute this tendency?

2. Using the principle cited in preceding question, describe how you would employ EMG biofeedback to promote muscular relaxation.

Massage Techniques

Objective

To understand and demonstrate the proper application procedures for the various types of massage techniques.

Materials Needed

- Massage lubricant
- Towels or sheets
- Blood pressure cuff and stethoscope
- Goniometer
- Tape measure

Procedures

1. **Traditional (Hoffa) massage**
   a. Position the patient in a comfortable and accessible position.
   b. Drape the area if necessary.
   c. Inspect the area for contraindications.
   d. Measure the patient's heart rate and blood pressure prior to beginning the treatments. Record this information on the chart provided. It is recommended that a third person in the laboratory group take pulse and blood pressure measurements throughout the treatment, thereby not interrupting the massage.
   e. Apply lubricant.
   f. Begin with light effleurage, and gradually build to deep effleurage.
   g. Begin pétrissage, and proceed into tapotement.
   h. When finished with tapotement, reapply pétrissage and then deep effleurage.
   i. Make sure to end the treatment with light effleurage.
   j. Record your patient's responses to the different phases of the treatment on the chart provided.
2. **Friction massage**
   a. Position the patient in a comfortable and relaxed position.
   b. Using a goniometer, measure the range of motion of the joint to be treated. Record this information on the chart provided.
   c. Begin by performing light circular strokes that run perpendicular or parallel to the underlying muscle tissue.
   d. Progress to firmer, deeper strokes. The amount of force applied must be enough to reach deep into the tissue.
   e. Record your patient's responses to the treatment.
3. **Myofascial release**
   a. Position the patient in a comfortable and relaxed position.
   b. Using a goniometer, measure the range of motion of the joint to be treated. Record this information on the chart provided.
   c. **J-strokes**
      i. Locate the adhesion.
      ii. Place one hand on the skin so that the adhesion is on stretch.
      iii. Using the 2nd and 3rd fingers of the other hand, stroke the skin in the opposite direction, ending in a curl (like the letter J).
      iv. Continue process until adhesions are reduced in size.
      v. Record your patient's responses to the treatment.
   d. **Focused stretching**
      i. Locate the affected area.
      ii. Place the heel of one hand in the affected area, and place the opposite arm crossed in front of the other arm. (Your hands should be pulling the area in opposite directions.)
      iii. Apply a stretch to the tissues, using a slow, deep pressure.
      iv. Repeat until there are no restrictions felt in the area.
      v. Record your patient's responses to the treatment.
   e. **Skin rolling**
      i. Begin by progressing from the inferior and lateral segment of the treated area, and progress medially and superiorly.
      ii. Lift and separate the tissue by using your thumb and fingers.

iii. Roll the skin between your fingers. Be sure to note any limitations.

iv. If and when you note an adhesion area:

1. Lift the skin, and move it in the direction of the restriction.
2. Move the skin in the direction of the restriction.
3. If the adhesion still persists, move the skin diagonally.
4. Repeat this process until the adhesions are resolved.

v. Repeat the entire process beginning at the superior and lateral portion of the body area, and proceed to the inferior medial portion.

vi. Record your patient's responses to the treatment.

f. **Arm pull/leg pull**

i. Position the patient supine with the arm relaxed at the side.

ii. Grasp the extremity at the thenar and hypothenar eminence or just proximal to the wrist.

iii. Apply a gentle traction force that is in line with the anterior deltoid.

iv. Hold the stretch until the arm feels relaxed.

v. Repeat the procedure with the arm abducted 10–15°. Continue the process until full abduction is achieved or glenohumeral pathology limits motion.

vi. Record your patient's responses to the treatment.

g. **Diagonal release**

i. This procedure will require two individuals.

ii. Have the patient lie prone or supine.

iii. One individual should grasp the leg just above

the ankle joint and the other grasps the opposite arm above the wrist.

iv. While maintaining the arm and leg horizontal to each other, one individual stabilizes the extremity while the other moves the limb until adhesions are felt. A gentle traction force is then applied.

v. Repeat the above step until all adhesions have been reduced.

vi. Repeat the process with the opposite limbs and also with the opposite clinician applying the stabilizing force.

vii. Record your patient's responses to the treatment.

4. **Edema reduction**

a. Mark two areas on the extremity to measure the circumference of the extremity in the area to be treated. Measure the circumference, and record it on the chart provided.

b. Elevate the body part to be treated.

c. Apply lubricant to the area.

d. Position yourself distal to the area to be treated.

e. Begin by making long, slow strokes toward the heart, starting proximal to the injured area. Every fourth or fifth stroke, move the starting point of the massage slightly distal.

f. Continue stroking the area longitudinally, and gradually move the starting point distally.

g. Once you reach the distal portion of the edematous area, begin to work back to your original starting point.

h. Remeasure the circumferences marked previously. Record your patient's responses to the treatment.

Massage Techniques

Name: _____ Date: _____

Subject(s): _____

Traditional massage			
	Heart Rate	**Blood Pressure**	**Sensations**
Pretreatment measurements			
Effleurage			
Pétrissage			
Tapotement			

Friction massage and myofascial release			
	Pretreatment ROM	**Post-treatment ROM**	**Sensations**
Friction			
Myofascial release: J-strokes			
Myofascial release: Focused stretching			
Myofascial release: Skin rolling			
Myofascial release: Arm pull/Leg pull			
Myofascial release: Diagonal release			

Edema reduction		
Measurement location	**Pretreatment measurement**	**Post-treatment measurement**
Proximal mark		
Distal mark		

▪ Activity Questions

1. Which of the massage techniques would you use to treat an athlete with bicipital tendonitis? Achilles tendonitis? Subacute ankle sprain?

2. Which of the myofascial techniques do you find to be most useful?

3. Why are there four suggested techniques for myofascial release? Compare and contrast the differences between each of the techniques.

4. What information should you record in the patient's file following the completion of a massage treatment?

Manual Traction: Cervical

Objective

To determine the effectiveness of manual cervical traction in improving range of motion, in reducing pain, and in reducing perceived muscle tension about the cervical spine.

Materials Needed

- Padded plinth
- Adjustable-height stool for the clinician
- Timing device
- Goniometer

Procedures

1. Determine and record the baseline measurements of cervical active range of motion.
2. Establish a 0–10 rating on pain and perceived tension in cervical musculature.
3. Position the patient supine near the edge of the plinth. Comfortably rest patient's head in the clinician's hands, and establish relaxation of the patient's musculature before proceeding.
4. Position the head and neck in approximately 10–20° of neck flexion.
5. Using fingertip pressure at the base of the skull, provide a light amount of traction force.
6. Establish comfort level of patient before proceeding with increasing levels of traction force.
7. Hold traction force up to 60 seconds, and repeat 3–5 times.
8. Reassess cervical range of motion, pain, and perceived musculature tension.

Notes

1. Perform the same procedures after the use of other modalities (e.g., superficial heating modalities) to increase relaxation.
2. If fingertip pressure is uncomfortable to the patient, use a more broad-handed grip to gain purchase (improved grip over a broader area) for traction force.
3. Alter the amount of neck flexion during the treatment to determine best line of pull.

Manual Traction: Cervical

Name: _____ Date: _____

Subject(s): _____

Range of motion	Pretreatment measurement	Post-treatment measurement
Flexion		
Extension		
Lateral flexion (right)		
Lateral flexion (left)		

■ Perceived Muscle Tension

Pretreatment measurement—perceived muscle tension:

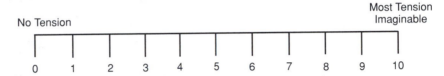

Post-treatment measurement—perceived muscle tension:

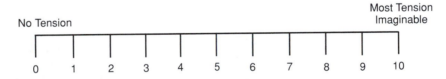

■ Activity Questions

1. Many patients have difficulty trusting their head in the hands of a relative stranger, especially in a painful situation. How can you establish this relaxation? Is traction beneficial if the patient is not able to relax?

2. Clinicians endure a grueling day of work regularly. It is not uncommon to face fatigue during the workday. Note the amount of energy required to perform manual traction. What are some ways that you can limit the amount of fatigue faced with manual traction?

Intermittent Mechanical Traction

Objective

To establish the effectiveness of intermittent lumbar and cervical mechanical traction on range of motion, pain, and perceived musculature tension.

Materials Needed

- Traction table (preferably friction-free settings) with adjustable height control
- Traction machine that intermittently applies pulling force
- Spreader bar with rope attached at end
- Thoracic harness that fits around the lower thoracic ribs below the xiphoid process
- Pelvic corset that fits snugly over the iliac crests
- Head halter fitting snugly at occiput and chin, or cervical traction ramp with adjusts at mastoid processes

Procedures

Establish baseline lumbar and/or cervical range of motion, pain rating (0–10 scale), and perceived musculature tension (0–10 scale).

Lumbar traction
1. Arrange the pelvic corset and the thoracic harness on the table in the position they will be placed on the patient.
2. Place the patient on the table in the desired position (the amount of flexion is determined by dysfunction). Place leg rest of pillows under knees to alter flexion angle.
3. Attach the lumbar corset first, then apply the thoracic harness, and let it overlap slightly to allow for the minor slippage that will occur during treatment. Fit both appliances snugly.
4. Attach the rope to the corset with the hook or the spreader bar.
5. Secure the thoracic harness to the table.
6. Select the amount of force, the on-off cycle, and the duration of the treatment. The parameters chosen must be within the patient's tolerance and comfort. Begin with a traction force approximately 25% of the patient's body weight.
7. Turn on the machine, and let it pull for a few seconds to remove the slack from the straps.
8. Release the table catch to allow for friction-free treatment.
9. Monitor patient for several cycles to ensure comfort. Provide the patient with the stop switch.
10. Re-assess lumbar range of motion, pain rating, and perceived lumbar musculature tension.

Cervical traction
1. Prepare the table with the head harness or cervical traction ramp. Adjust the angulation of the rope or ramp for the specific dysfunction. Place a pillow under the knees to promote relaxation.
2. Position the patient, and adjust the halter or ramp.
3. Attach the ramp or halter to the spreader bar. The rope must be slack to attach the spreader bar, but the slack should be removed before the treatment.
4. Select the force, the duration of the on-off cycle, and the duration of the treatment. The suggested amount of force to use initially is 10–15 pounds. Then increase the force to achieve the desired amount of pull the patient can tolerate.
5. Turn on the machine, and make certain that the pull the patient experiences comes from the occiput.
6. Monitor the patient for several cycles to ensure comfort. Provide the patient with the stop switch.
7. Re-assess cervical range of motion, pain rating, and perceived cervical musculature tension.

Notes

1. The on-off cycle, the amount of pull, and the angle of pull may need to be altered to determine most effective treatment.
2. Other relation-inducing modalities may be used prior to the traction treatment.

Intermittent Mechanical Traction

Name: _____   Date: _____

Subject(s): _____

Lumbar traction		
Range of motion	**Pretreatment measurement**	**Post-treatment measurement**
Flexion		
Extension		
Lateral flexion (right)		
Lateral flexion (left)		

■ Perceived Muscle Tension

Pretreatment Measurement—perceived muscle tension:

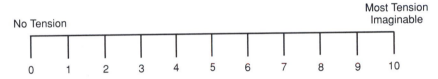

Post-treatment Measurement—perceived muscle tension:

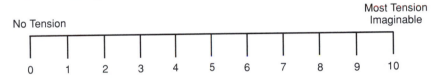

Cervical traction		
Range of Motion	**Pretreatment measurement**	**Post-treatment measurement**
Flexion		
Extension		
Lateral flexion (right)		
Lateral flexion (left)		

■ Perceived Muscle Tension

Pretreatment Measurement—perceived muscle tension:

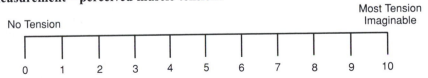

Post-treatment Measurement—perceived muscle tension:

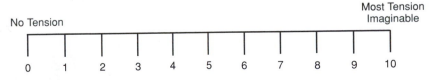

▪ Activity Questions

1. Why is the friction-free traction table so important for lumbar traction? Can traction be implemented effectively without the traction table?

2. If your patient is concerned about the force that will be applied during traction, what measures can you take to prepare your patient for the treatment session? If your patient appears extremely tense about the treatment should you continue with it?

Supine vs. Sitting Cervical Traction

■ Objective

To determine the effects of gravity on the force needed for cervical traction.

■ Materials Needed

- Cervical traction unit
- 20-lb weight and an assortment of other free weights

■ Procedures

1. Attach the rope from the traction unit to the 20-lb weight, allowing the weight to rest freely from the unit.
2. If a mechanical traction unit is being used, turn it on. If a pulley system is being used, begin to add weight in measurable increments
3. Gradually increase the tension until the weight begins to rise. Record the tension at the point where the weight is first lifted from the table (Fig. 6–4).
4. Reposition the traction unit so that the weight will be pulled across the table (Fig. 6–5). Gradually increase the tension until the weight begins to slide. Record this value on the chart provided.
5. Repeat Steps 1 through 5 using different weights.

■ Notes

- If a commercial traction unit is not available, this activity can be performed using a rope and free weights in 1- and 2-lb increments.
- In this activity, the 20-lb weight approximates the weight of the human head. The effects of gravity become apparent in the increased load necessary to lift rather than slide the weight. The therapeutic effects of cervical traction will not be realized until the forces of gravity are overcome. For this reason, cervical traction applied in the supine position is preferred over cervical traction in the sitting position. The benefit of encouraging muscle relaxation is also added when the person is supine.

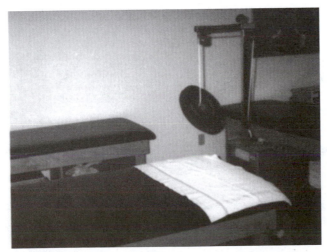

Figure 6–4. Set-up of traction unit with weight lifted off the table.

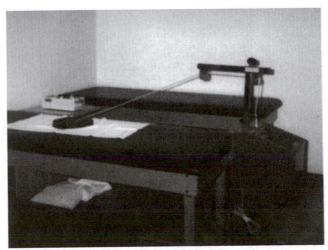

Figure 6–5. Set-up of traction unit with weight sliding across the table.

Supine vs. Sitting Cervical Traction

Name: _____   Date: _____

Subject(s): _____

Weight	Force Required		Force Required		
	Vertical	Horizontal	Vertical	Horizontal	% Difference
20 lb.					

▪ Activity Questions

1. What was the difference between the amount of tension required to raise the weight vertically compared with the amount of tension required to slide the weight across the table? Did this percentage remain constant when other weights were used?

2. What other factors account for the amount of tension required to slide the weight across the table?

Continuous Passive Motion

Objective

To determine the effectiveness of continuous passive motion (CPM) in maintaining range of motion to prevent the negative effects of immobilization.

Materials Needed

- Padded plinth
- CPM unit
- Tape measure
- Goniometer

Procedures

1. Ensure the patient does not have contraindication to the use of CPM.
2. Position the patient for comfort on the plinth.
3. Measure the length of the extremity to be placed in the CPM unit. For example, if using a lower extremity CPM unit, measure the length of the thigh (ischial tuberosity to knee joint line) and the lower leg (knee joint line to approximately $\frac{1}{4}$ inch below the heel). Record these measurements.
4. Place the extremity into the CPM unit.
5. Adjust the length of the unit for the extremity.
6. Attach the restraining straps, ensuring they are not too tight.
7. Instruct the patient on the use of the hand-held control to change the speed of the movement or stop movement.
8. Select an appropriate speed (rate at which the CPM moves) for the treatment. Record this information in the patient's record.
9. Set the range of motion of the CPM unit to what was prescribed by the physician. Record the range of motion for the treatment in the patient's record.
10. Look for pressure sites on the patient caused by the CPM unit, and make adjustments as necessary.
11. Set the time for the treatment. For purposes of this laboratory activity, the treatment time will be 5 minutes.
12. At the end of the treatment, remove the restraining straps; lift the extremity from the CPM unit.
13. Check the extremity for pressure sores and other signs/symptoms of inflammation, compartmental pressure, or DVT. Record the patient's tolerance to the treatment.

Notes

- Different types of CPM devices require slightly different set-up procedures. Please refer to manufacturer's specifications for proper use.
- In addition to the range of motion and treatment speed measurements, a pain scale may be used to record pre- and post-treatment pain levels.

Continuous Passive Motion

Name: _____   Date: _____

Subject(s): _____

CPM and Patient Information	
Extremity measurement	
Speed of treatment	
Treatment ROM	
Patient response	

▉ Activity Questions

1. In general, CPM treatments progress from a limited range of motion to full range of motion. What indications would you look for to address the rate of increasing range of motion in successive treatments? What signs or symptoms might suggest you are progressing the range of motion too quickly?

2. When using a CPM device for a postsurgical patient, you must check for signs of intracompartmental pressures and DVT. What are these signs?

On completion of the activities for Unit 6, review the following case studies to enhance practical application of mechanical modalities.

1. You have a basketball player who has sustained a Grade 2 lateral ankle sprain. The possibility of fracture has been ruled out. His ankle has significant post-traumatic edema. Develop a treatment protocol for the first 3 days postinjury.

2. A 57-year-old assembly-line worker comes to you to get help in relieving pain and muscle spasms of the neck and upper back region. A thorough assessment reveals cervical nerve root impingement. One of the modalities you decide to use to treat this patient is traction. What type of traction will you use? Why? How will you position this patient for the treatment?

3. A soccer player reports to your clinic 3 weeks after he sprained his ankle. He reports having sprained this ankle before. He states that the post-trauma radiographs were negative for fractures. He did not follow up with rehabilitation for the sprain, stating that he thought he could take care of this ankle injury just as he had cared for his previous ankle sprains. He is frustrated that it is 3 weeks postinjury and that he still has swelling and a slight decrease in dorsiflexion range of motion. What can you do to attempt to eliminate the remaining swelling and increase range of motion?

Appendix A

Methods to Monitor Skin Surface Temperature

The ideal method of monitoring the surface temperature of the skin during and after application of thermal modalities is using an electronic sensor specifically designed for this purpose. These devices have a special sensor in their tips that allows them to measure temperature rapidly and accurately. Their output is displayed with either an analog meter or a more accurate digital readout.

These meters are not ordinary items and may not be found in many educational settings. The following devices have been used in place of these more "high-tech" devices.

■ Electronic Outdoor Thermometer

Digital outdoor thermometers (those possessing wire leads) may be used to accurately measure changes in skin temperature. We recommend placing the sensor on the skin and then covering it with a 2×3–inch piece of Neoprene material (cut from an old knee sleeve) during the temperature reading (Fig. A). Experimentation is needed with individual units to determine the amount of time required to read the temperature change fully. Advantages of this type of unit include accuracy by way of a digital readout, and some units have memories in which temperature readings may be stored. Radio Shack has a line of electronic thermometers, with costs ranging $15–$30.

■ General Instructions

With either instrument, remove the Neoprene covering when temperatures are not being taken so that the cooling or warming process is not incorrectly influenced.

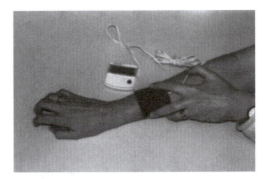

Figure A.   Placement of thermometer.

Appendix B

Interfacing Electrical Modalities with an Oscilloscope

A standard oscilloscope can be used to see the actual pulse form generated by various electrical modalities in various modes. As presented in Figure 18, two leads, one of the oscilloscope's active leads and its reference lead, are spliced into one of the cables exiting the generator. The other active lead is connected to the cable of the modality. A 100- to 2000-ohm (Ω) resistor (available from an electronics supply store) is connected between the terminal ends of each of the modality's cables to roughly represent skin resistance. The oscilloscope's input parameters (e.g., amperage threshold and sweep rate) are then adjusted to the particular modality and its output parameters.

After making the connections described above, turn on the oscilloscope and the modality. Fine-tune the display so that the pulse's baseline is centered on the oscilloscope's grid, and make other fine-tuning adjustments as required. Modify the modality's output parameters, and note the corresponding changes on the oscilloscope. When the output intensity is increased or decreased, the height (amplitude) of the pulse will change correspondingly; increasing the pulse duration will cause the pulse to widen; increasing the number of pulses per second will increase the number of pulses displayed on the screen. Change modalities, and notice the similarities and differences in the pulse shapes.

The benefits of this demonstration are largely dependent on the type of oscilloscope being used. Many advanced models have options to freeze the screen, and others provide for printing the current image.

Assistance with the materials needed for this project are often available through an engineering or a physics department.

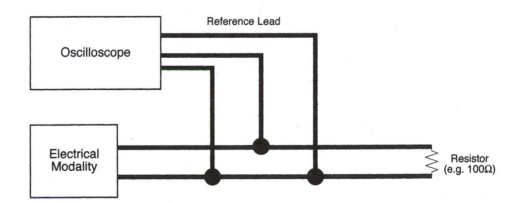

References

1. Buyag, R: The cooling, analgesic, and rewarming effects of ice massage on localized skin. Physical Therapy 55:11, 1975.
2. Weinberger, A and Lev, A: Temperature elevation of connective tissue by physical modalities. Critical Reviews in Physical Rehabilitation Medicine 3:121, 1991.
3. Palmer, JE and Knight, KL: Ankle and thigh skin surface temperature changes with repeated ice pack application. Journal of Athletic Training 31:319, 1996.
4. Watkins, MP: Clinical evaluation of thermal agents. In Michlovitz, SL (ed): Thermal Agents in Rehabilitation, ed. 2. FA Davis, Philadelphia, 1990, pp 221–244.
5. Arnheim, DD and Prentice, WE: Principles of Athletic Training, ed. 8. Mosby, St. Louis, 1993, pp 308–346.
6. Ingersoll, CD and Mangus, BC: Sensations of cold re-examined: A study using the McGill Pain Questionnaire. Journal of Athletic Training 26:240, 1991.
7. Streator, S, Ingersoll, CD and Knight, KL: Sensory information can decrease cold-induced pain perception. Journal of Athletic Training 30:293, 1995.
8. Evans, TA et al: Agility following the application of cold therapy. Journal of Athletic Training 30:231, 1995.
9. Cross, KM, et al: Functional performance following an ice immersion to the lower extremity. Journal of Athletic Training 31:113, 1996.
10. Kimura, IF et al: The effect of cryotherapy on eccentric plantar flexion peak torque and endurance. Journal of Athletic Training 32:124, 1997.
11. Thieme, HA, et al: Cooling does not affect knee proprioception. Journal of Athletic Training 31:8, 1996.
12. DeLitto, A and Rose, SJ: Comparative comfort of three waveforms used in electrically eliciting quadriceps femoris muscle contractions. Physical Therapy 66:1704, 1986.
13. Nelson, RM and Currier, DP: Electrical stimulation of healthy muscle and tissue repair. In Nelson, RM and Currier, DP (eds): Clinical Electrotherapy, ed. 2. Appleton & Lange, Norwalk, CT, 1991, pp 106–107.
14. Miller, CR and Webers, RL: The effects of ice massage on an individual's pain tolerance level to electrical stimulation. JOSPT 12:105, 1990.
15. Durst, JW, et al.: Effects of ice and recovery time on maximal involuntary isometric torque production using electrical stimulation. JOSPT 13:240, 1991.
16. Robinson, AJ: Instrumentation in electrotherapy. In Robinson, AJ and Snyder-Mackler, L: Clinical Electrophysiology. Williams & Wilkins, Baltimore, 1995, p 73.
17. Cameron, MH and Monroe, LG: Relative transmission of ultrasound by media customarily used for phonophoresis. Physical Therapy 72:142, 1992.
18. Klucinec, B: The effectiveness of the Aquaflex gel pad in the transmission of acoustic energy. Journal of Athletic Training 31:313, 1996.
19. Belitsky, RB, Odam, SJ and Hubley-Kozey, C: Evaluation of the effectiveness of wet ice, dry ice, and cryogen packs in reducing skin temperature. Physical Therapy 67:1080, 1987.
20. Bocobo, C et al: The effect of ice on intra-articular temperature in the knee of the dog. American Journal of Physical Medicine and Rehabilitation 70:181, 1991.
21. Michlovitz, SL: Cryotherapy: The use of cold as a therapeutic agent. In Michlovitz, SL (ed): Thermal Agents in Rehabilitation, ed. 2. FA Davis, Philadelphia, 1990, pp 63–84.
22. Nimchick, PSR and Knight, KL: Effects of wearing a toe cap or sock on temperature and perceived pain during ice immersion. Journal of Athletic Training 18:144, 1983.
23. Ingersoll, CD and Mangus, BC: Habituation to the perception of the qualities of cold-induced pain. Journal of Athletic Training 27:218, 1992.
24. Tsang, KKW: The effects of cryotherapy applied through various barriers. Journal of Sports Rehabilitation 6:343, 1997.
25. Malone, TR: Nerve injury in athletes caused by cryotherapy. Journal of Athletic Training 27:235, 1992.
26. Minton, J: A comparison of thermotherapy and cryotherapy in enhancing supine, extended-leg hip flexion. Journal of Athletic Training 28:172, 1993.
27. Lentell, G, et al: The use of thermal agents to influence the effectiveness of a low-load prolonged stretch. JOSPT 16:200, 1992.
28. Myrer JW, Measom G, and Fellingham GW: Temperature changes in the human leg during and after two methods of cryotherapy. Journal of Athletic Training 33: 1998, 25.
29. DeLitto, A and Robinson, AJ: Electrical stimulation of muscle: Techniques and applications. In Snyder-Mackler, L and Robinson, AJ (eds): Clinical Electrophysiology: Electrotherapy and Electrophysiologic Testing. Williams & Wilkins, Baltimore, 1989, p 102.

30. Hooker, DN: Electrical stimulating currents. In Prentice, W (ed): Therapeutic Modalities in Sports Medicine. Times Mirror/Mosby, St. Louis, 1990, p 61.

31. DeLitto, A and Robinson, AJ: Electrical stimulation of muscle: Techniques and applications. In Snyder-Mackler, L and Robinson, AJ (eds): Clinical Electrophysiology: Electrotherapy and Electrophysiologic Testing. Williams & Wilkins, Baltimore, 1989, p 101.

32. Mathews, J: The effects of spinal traction. Physiotherapy 58:64, 1972.

33. Tekeoglu, I, et al: Distraction of lumbar vertebrae in gravitational traction. Spine 23:1061, 1998.